SYNDROME IDENTIFICATION
for
Speech-Language Pathologists

AN ILLUSTRATED POCKETGUIDE

Robert J. Shprintzen, Ph.D.

Professor and Director
Communication Disorders Unit
Center for the Diagnosis, Study, and Treatment
of Velo-Cardio-Facial Syndrome
Center for Genetic Communication Disorders
Department of Otolaryngology and Communication Science
State University of New York Health Science Center
Syracuse, New York

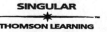
SINGULAR

THOMSON LEARNING

Africa • Australia • Canada • Denmark • Japan • Mexico • New Zealand • Philippines
Puerto Rico • Singapore • Spain • United Kingdom • United States

COPYRIGHT © 2000 Delmar. Singular Publishing Group is an imprint of Delmar, a division of Thomson Learning. Thomson Learning™ is a trademark used herein under license.

Printed in Canada
    XXX

For more information, contact Singular Publishing Group, 401 West "A" Street, Suite 325 San Diego, CA 92101-7904; or find us on the World Wide Web at http://www.singpub.com

Library of Congress Cataloging-in-Publication Data
Shprintzen, Robert J.
    Syndrome identification for speech-language pathologists :
Illustrated pocket guide / by Robert J. Shprintzen.
    p.   cm.
    Includes bibliographical references and index.
    ISBN 0-7693-0019-7 (soft cover : alk. paper)
    1. Syndromes Handbooks, manuales, etc. 2. Genetic disorders
Handbooks, manuals, etc. 3. Speech therapists Handbooks, manuals,
etc. I. Title.
    RC69.S48 2000   99-40684
                                      CIP

Contents

Syndromes With Speech, Language and Cognitive Impairments

Preface

The study of abnormalities of human morphology is not new. In centuries past, the focus was on the oddities of human malformations because the unusual in appearance and function have always fascinated humankind. Many ancient myths have been centered on abnormal appearance, from the ancient Egyptian god Bes who had all of the features of an individual with achondroplasia to the Greek cyclops who demonstrated the severe malformations associated with holoprosencephaly. In more modern times, most notably the 19th and early 20th century, freak shows were common forms of entertainment in traveling carnivals, featuring conjoined twins, individuals with hypertrichosis (excessive body and facial hair), and other malformations. Perhaps the most famous of human oddities during his time was Joseph Merrick, the Elephant Man, who is discussed briefly in this PocketGuide under the entry for Proteus syndrome. Fortunately, our study of human anomalies has evolved, as has our choice of entertainment. Beginning in the latter half of the 20th century, clinicians and scientists began to understand that the study of malformations could lead to a mechanism for relieving the suffering of people who had disorders that impaired the quantity or quality of life.

In the earliest years of study, individuals who studied human anomalies were called "syndromologists" or "teratologists" (from the Greek *teratos*, or monster). Today, the term *dysmorphologist* is more likely to be applied to those who diagnose individuals with malformations. Although some medical specialists do receive special postgraduate training in the field of clinical or medical genetics and may become board certified in these areas, the diagnosis of children with multiple anomaly syndromes is not discipline specific, nor do dysmorphologists come exclusively from medicine. The participation in the diagnostic process and the identification of multiple anomaly disorders can occur at any point in the process of providing clinical care. Because, by definition, multiple anomalies affect many different aspects of structure or function, many different clinicians should be able to recognize and diagnose conditions that intersect their area of professional study. The speech-language pathologist is no different.

There are quite literally thousands and thousands of conditions that involve multiple anomalies. Therefore, it would be impossible to list more than a small percentage of multiple anomaly disorders (syndromes) in this PocketGuide. For example, the *Online Mendelian Inheritance in Man* (or OMIM), an Internet site that lists and describes genetic conditions currently has over 10,000 entries. OMIM lists disorders of genetic etiology. There are many more disorders that are caused by teratogens or mechanical disruptions not listed in OMIM. Therefore, this PocketGuide lists a sampling of disorders that speech-language pathologists are likely to encounter regardless of their venue of practice. Although many of the disorders described are rare, because they present with communication disorders, they will certainly all be encountered by a speech-language pathologist somewhere.

Each entry is structured to provide a brief description of the types of communicative impairments that occur in association with the syndrome (speech production, voice, language, resonance, and hearing) as well as feeding disorders. These descriptions are, in most cases, based on the author's own observations and clinical experience together with the known phenotypic spectrum of the syndrome. Extensive descriptions of communicative impairments do not exist for most syndromes and it is hoped that this volume will ignite the interest of clinicians to contribute to the process of syndrome delineation. Also listed in each entry is the etiology of the disorder as currently understood and a comprehensive list of the anomalies associated with the syndrome. It is possible that some of the terms used to describe anomalies associated with the entries are unfamiliar to the reader. It is suggested that readers should utilize this PocketGuide as a road map to the world of multiple anomaly syndromes and that they continue to refer to other sources for additional information.

One caveat is offered regarding the etiologies listed. The study of genetically based syndromes is progressing at an unprecedented rate. The Human Genome Project has spurred an incredibly vigorous response to the study of human genetics and it is likely that a substantial amount of new information will be developed after the publication of this text. Every effort has been made to keep this information as current as possible, but new genes are being discovered on a daily basis. Again, readers are urged to pursue their interest in genetics by referring to the Internet, OMIM, and professional publications.

Acknowledgments

This is the fourth text that I have written or edited, so I have had the opportunity to acknowledge and thank my family, friends, and colleagues in previous volumes. To repeat these acknowledgments would trivialize them, and so I will not. Therefore, I would prefer to mention people who at one time or another were my students, because they have inspired me no less than those who handed knowledge down to me. I have had the opportunity to teach large classes, small seminars, but more frequently, my attempts to educate have been one-on-one with graduate students, postgraduate students, residents, and fellows. I have had the true pleasure of supervising or helping to guide more than 40 theses or research projects and many of my students have honored me with coauthorship of their papers published in peer-reviewed journals. Their names are really too numerous to mention, as are their professions, including speech-language pathologists, pediatricians, geneticists, otolaryngologists, plastic surgeons, and dental specialists. Today I call them names such as Karen and Tony, and they have long ago shed the practice of calling me "Dr. Shprintzen" and now call me Bob. They live in the U.S., Mexico, South America, Europe, and Asia and have been often invited me to visit, allowing me to observe the fruits of my tutelage in their own institutions. Several have become close colleagues; most have remained good friends. Whatever measure of knowledge I have imparted to them, they have more than returned to me many times over. I want them to understand that there is no greater honor for a teacher than to be taught by a student. I want them to know that I hold them all in the highest regard. They have truly served to validate my ideas and hypotheses and in so doing have demonstrated that my faith in them was justified and earned.

How to Use This PocketGuide

The syndromes listed in this guide represent a group of disorders that will be encountered by speech-language pathologists because they result in disorders of speech, language, cognition, or feeding. The symptoms listed for each entry, although comprehensive, may not necessarily be entirely complete, simply because the continued study of rare disorders results in new discoveries over time. Furthermore, if a symptom is listed, this does not mean that an individual case will definitely express this problem. Each entry lists *possible* anomalies associated with the syndrome, and in some cases *probable* findings, but none are obligatory. However, the listing may present readers with problem areas that they may wish to check if they were not previously suspected. For example, some disorders listed in this PocketGuide have late-onset or progressive disorders that may not be suspected when individual cases are seen at a very young age.

The entries are listed in alphabetical order according to the nosology preferred by the author. The reader should be aware that many syndromes have more than one label, and the clinician may be more familiar with the other appellation. For example, Down syndrome may also be labeled as trisomy 21. Velo-cardio-facial has been called DiGeorge syndrome, CATCH 22, and conotruncal anomalies face syndrome. Because of these differences in the naming of various syndromes, alternative labels are also provided.

The natural history of each entry is also described. This refers to the expected course of the disorder over time. Clinicians should be aware that multiple anomaly disorders are rarely static in their presentation. Therefore, an individual clinician's experience with a specific disorder may be limited by the age of the case he or she has encountered. The presentation of Prader-Willi syndrome is a good example. Many young children with Prader-Willi syndrome have hypernasal resonance, but this problem often resolves with age so that in adolescence, hypernasality may no longer be present. Therefore, one's experience with Prader-Willi syndrome in a pediatric setting will be different than for someone in an adult care facility. The clinician may wish to use these descriptions as a way of anticipating problems that may not have arisen as yet.

Aarskog Syndrome

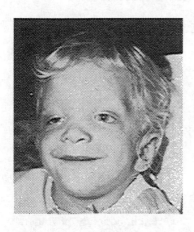

Aarskog syndrome: Note the unilateral upper eyelid ptosis and low set ears.

Also Known As: Faciogenital dysplasia; facial-digital-genital syndrome; faciodigitogenital syndrome; Aarskog-Scott syndrome

Aarskog syndrome is a syndrome characterized by short stature with other clinical features that are relatively subtle and may therefore be somewhat difficult to recognize. Some of the clinical manifestations, especially with regard to genital anomalies, become less obvious after puberty, which makes the diagnosis more difficult. As an X-linked recessive disorder, complete expression is typically seen in males with minor manifestations in mothers who are carriers. Many cases have been described in the medical literature, but the syndrome is probably relatively rare with birth incidence estimated to be approximately 1:100,000.

Major System(s) Affected: Craniofacial; limbs; growth; genitourinary; musculoskeletal.

Etiology: X-linked recessive inheritance caused by a mutation in the FGD1 gene mapped to Xp11.21.

Speech Disorders: Speech may be marked by obligatory articulation of anterior sounds secondary to dental spacing anomalies and congenitally missing teeth that do not typically interfere with intelligibility. Lingual protrusion may occur secondary to missing anterior teeth, or lateralization secondary to missing lateral incisors or premolars. Cleft lip and/or palate occurs occasionally in the syndrome and may result in the speech disorders commonly associated with clefting (hypernasality and articulation disorders).

Feeding Disorders: None have been reported or observed.

Hearing Disorders: Hearing loss is not a feature of Aarskog syndrome, but in cases with cleft palate, middle ear effusion, and transient conductive loss is possible.

Voice Disorders: There are no known voice disorders associated with Aarskog syndrome.

Resonance Disorders: In cases with clefts, there may be hypernasal resonance. Otherwise, resonance is within normal limits.

Language Disorders: Borderline normal intellect or mild cognitive impairment is a common feature of Aarskog syndrome, and mild language delay and impairment often results. However, the majority of patients with Aarskog syndrome tend to have normal language and speech onset.

Other Clinical Features:

Craniofacial: orbital hypertelorism; wide palpebral fissures; ptosis; short nose with anteverted nostrils and a wide nasal tip;

Limbs: mild soft tissue syndactyly of the fingers and toes (mild webbing); broad toes; abnormal terminal and middle phalanges of the fingers; clinodactyly of fingers and toes; digital contractures;

Growth: short stature; delayed bone age;

Genitourinary: shawled or bifid scrotum; cryptorchidism;

Musculoskeletal: inguinal hernia; cervical spine anomalies including spina bifida occulta, vertebral fusions, and hypoplasia of the odontoid process.

Natural History: Growth deficiency is postnatal in onset and may not be detected until later in childhood. The digital and dental anomalies also become more pronounced with age. The facial abnormalities are also typically mild and may go undetected, possibly resulting in underdetection of this syndrome.

Treatment Prognosis: The prognosis for resolution of the speech disorders associated with this syndrome is excellent, and general prognosis is also excellent.

Differential Diagnosis: The facial appearance and short stature resemble **Noonan syndrome,** and the facial and digital anomalies may resemble **otopalatodigital syndrome, type I.** Both Noonan and OPD type I also have mild cognitive impairment as a feature. Aarskog syndrome should also be differentiated from other syndromes with postnatal onset of short stature that have craniofacial, limb, or genital anomalies. **Robinow syndrome** has a somewhat similar facial appearance, hypertelorism, occasional cleft lip and/or palate, genital anomalies in males, shortening of the limbs, and clinodactyly.

Aase-Smith Syndrome

Also Known As: Aase-Smith I syndrome

This is a rare syndrome with neurological manifestations that may be incompatible with life in many patients. Therefore, it is unusual to find surviving adults or older children. However, neonates with multiple joint contractures and failure-to-thrive should be suspected of having Aase-Smith syndrome, prompting referral for neurologic evaluation and possible MR or CT scan.

Major System(s) Affected: Central nervous system; craniofacial; limbs; cardiac.

Etiology: Autosomal dominant inheritance. The gene has not been identified or mapped as yet.

Speech Disorders: Various degrees of articulatory impairment should be expected based on three factors: the extent of central nervous system involvement; presence of cleft palate; the degree of limitation of oral opening. Dysarthric and neurologically impaired speech may occur secondary to hydrocephalus or Dandy-Walker anomaly. Clefting of the palate is common and may result in compensatory articulation patterns. Further complicating both of these issues is the presence of multiple joint contractures, including the temporomandibular joint which may limit oral opening severely.

Feeding Disorders: Feeding in infancy may be severely impaired by both limited oral opening and severe neurologic disorders caused by Dandy-Walker anomaly. In the most severe cases, failure-to-thrive is to be expected. Cleft palate may complicate feeding, but it is of minimal importance in children with Aase-Smith syndrome. The neurologic and oral-opening disorders contribute far more to the feeding problems.

Hearing Disorders: Conductive hearing loss related to middle ear effusion and minor malformations of the external auditory canal should be expected.

Voice Disorders: Voice disorders have not been reported in association with Aase-Smith syndrome.

Resonance Disorders: Hypernasality should be anticipated in individuals with clefts, and may be exacerbated by limited oral opening which will decrease oral resonance.

Language Disorders: Language impairment may range from mild to severe, depending on the severity of the central nervous system anomalies.

Other Clinical Features:

Central nervous system: Dandy-Walker anomaly; hydrocephalus; neuroblastoma;

Craniofacial: cleft palate; limited oral opening; malformed auricles; ptosis;

Limbs: joint contractures; absent knuckles; digital contractures; club foot (talipes equinovarus);

Cardiac: heart malformations including ventriculoseptal defect.

Natural History: Some children with Aase-Smith syndrome are stillborn or die shortly after birth because of the severity of central nervous system involvement. In those who survive, there is no significant progression of the disorder, including the contractures and neurologic effects.

Treatment Prognosis: In the most severely affected individuals, the prognosis is very poor which is dependent on the degree of central nervous system malformation. In milder expressions, each disorder can be treated symptomatically with potentially good outcome.

Differential Diagnosis: Joint contractures and cleft palate are commonly seen in **distal arthrogryposis syndrome** which also has limited oral opening as a feature. **Christian syndrome** is characterized by contractures, cleft palate, early feeding disorders, and severe central nervous system anomalies. Early death is typical in **Christian syndrome**. **Pena-Shokeir syndrome** is also characterized by joint contractures, craniofacial anomalies, and early death. **Aicardi syndrome** also has contractures with Dandy-Walker anomaly, as well as clefting of the lip and palate.

Abruzzo-Erickson Syndrome

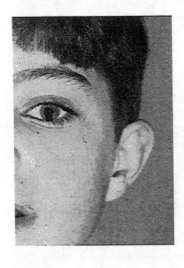

Iris coloboma is one of the major anomalies associated with Abruzzo-Erikson syndrome.

Also Known As:

This rare syndrome of hearing impairment (primarily sensorineural) also features craniofacial anomalies including cleft palate. The communicative phenotype can be confusing because the effects of the hearing impairment are superimposed on the resonance disorders that may accompany cleft palate. The presence of an ocular coloboma (cleft of the iris) may lead clinicians to suspect that patients with Abruzzo-Erickson syndrome have *CHARGE association.*

Major System(s) Affected:

Craniofacial; growth; ocular; genital; musculoskeletal.

Etiology:

X-linked recessive inheritance. The gene has not yet been identified or mapped.

Speech Disorders:

Speech may be affected by the hearing loss associated with Abruzzo-Erickson syndrome, and articulation may also be impaired from the effects of velopharyngeal insufficiency secondary to cleft palate.

Feeding Disorders: Other than the early effect of cleft palate, feeding is unaffected.

Hearing Disorders: Hearing loss is typically mixed with a major sensorineural component.

Voice Disorders: None.

Resonance Disorders: Resonance may be affected by velopharyngeal insufficiency secondary to cleft palate and may be exacerbated by hearing loss if the sensorineural component is severe.

Language Disorders: Expressive language is only affected if the sensorineural component of the hearing loss is severe.

Other Clinical Features:

Craniofacial: cleft palate; large, soft auricles;

Growth: short stature;

Ocular: ocular coloboma;

Genital: hypospadias;

Musculoskeletal: radial synostosis.

Natural History: The anomalies in Abruzzo-Erikson syndrome are essentially static except for the hearing loss. The sensorineural component of the hearing loss may be progressive in some patients.

Treatment Prognosis: Intellect is normal and the general prognosis for normal speech and language is good depending on the severity of the sensorineural component of the hearing loss.

Differential Diagnosis: At the time the syndrome was delineated, there was speculation that Abruzzo-Erickson syndrome actually represented **CHARGE association.** However, there is no doubt that this condition is distinct from **CHARGE.**

Achondroplasia

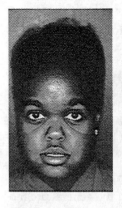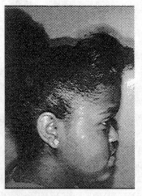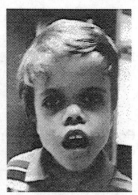

Achondroplasia: Note the midface deficiency and depressed nasal root. In the case shown at far right, note the chronic open-mouth posture indicative of upper airway obstruction.

Also Known As:

Achondroplasia is probably the most easily recognized genetic syndrome of short stature, especially short stature associated with disproportionately short limbs. The majority of cases are new mutations, but once the mutation has occurred, it is inherited as an autosomal dominant syndrome. Because there are many marriages between people of short stature, there have been homozygous cases (babies who have inherited two copies of the mutant gene, one from each parent). Homozygotes do not survive the more severe expression of the syndrome. Achondroplasia is a fairly common genetic disorder with a population prevalence of approximately 1:16,000 to 1:30,000. The exact frequency is somewhat difficult to calculate because other syndromes of short stature often resemble achondroplasia, and in the past, the diagnosis was applied inappropriately because of the lumping together of several different disorders.

Major System(s) Affected:

Growth; limbs; craniofacial.

Etiology: Autosomal dominant inheritance caused by a mutation in the FGFR3 gene (fibroblast growth factor receptor 3) mapped to 4p16.3. The majority of cases represent new spontaneous mutations.

Speech Disorders: Articulation impairment secondary to anterior skeletal open-bite is common in achondroplasia. In cases with neurologic impairment secondary to hydrocephalus, there may be some neurologically based articulation impairment.

Feeding Disorders: Early airway compromise may contribute to failure-to-thrive. In later life, obesity is common.

Hearing Disorders: Conductive hearing impairment is common related to chronic middle ear effusion. Sensorineural hearing loss has been reported in a small percentage of cases.

Voice Disorders: Hoarseness is common in achondroplasia, and may be related to ossification of the laryngeal cartilages. Laryngeal position is also abnormal because of skull base anomalies.

Resonance Disorders: Hyponasality is very common in achondroplasia related to chronic nasopharyngeal obstruction. Abnormal oral resonance may also occur secondary to tonsillar obstruction of the oropharynx. The tonsils may be of normal size, but the entire pharyngeal airway is abnormally configured in achondroplasia so that the tonsils are often abnormally positioned.

Language Disorders: Language development is usually normal unless there are secondary neurologic complications from hydrocephalus.

Other Clinical Features:

Growth: severe short stature (mean adult height is approximately 50 to 52 inches); osteochondrodysplasia; short limbs and digits (rhizomelic shortening); large head circumference; severe lordosis of the spine;

Limbs: restricted flexion of the elbows and hips;

Craniofacial: broad, prominent forehead; hydrocephalus; compression of the brain stem caused by abnormal stenosis of the foramen magnum; depressed nasal root;

severe shortening of the anterior cranial base; cranial base kyphosis; strabismus.

Natural History: Although the manifestations of achondroplasia are obvious at birth, growth deficiency becomes more pronounced with age and the body more disproportionate to the limbs. Progressive stenosis of the foramen magnum can cause compression of the brain stem and spinal cord. Obstructive sleep apnea may become evident in late childhood or early adolescence, even if upper airway obstruction has not been noted in infancy. Obesity is common, which may exacerbate the obstructive sleep apnea.

Treatment Prognosis: The articulation impairment seen in achondroplasia is related to the skeletal anomalies of the cranial base that result in abnormal position and angulation of the lower jaw in relation to a short and hypoplastic maxilla. The articulation errors are obligatory in nature and will not typically resolve with speech therapy alone. However, orthognathic or craniofacial surgery may correct the anomaly and the articulation impairment may resolve spontaneously or with some speech therapy after surgery. The neurologic manifestations of the syndrome also require surgical intervention.

Differential Diagnosis: There are many syndromes with disproportionate shortening of the limbs in relation to a more normal trunk size, including pseudoachondroplasia, achondrogenesis, **diastrophic dysplasia, hypochondroplasia,** and **Ellis-van Creveld syndrome.**

Acrocallosal Syndrome

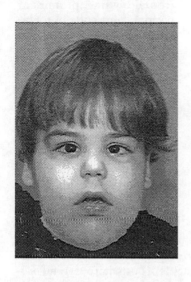

Acrocallosal syndrome: note depressed nasal root and strabismus.

Also Known As: Schinzel syndrome, ACLS

Acrocallosal syndrome was first delineated by Swiss geneticist Albert Schinzel in 1979. Although a rare disorder, it has sufficient overlap with other multiple anomaly disorders that some cases may have been misdiagnosed. Severe cognitive impairment is the rule and many patients do not develop intelligible speech.

Major System(s) Affected: Central nervous system; limbs and digits; craniofacial; cardiac; genitals; growth; abdominal.

Etiology: Autosomal recessive inheritance, mapped to the short arm of chromosome 12.

Speech Disorders: Many individuals with acrocallosal syndrome do not develop intelligible speech because of severe cognitive impairment. Cleft lip and palate occurs in over 10% of cases, which may further impair speech intelligibility.

Feeding Disorders: Severe hypotonia in infancy may result in a poor suck, but no other problems have been reported.

Hearing Disorders: Sensorineural hearing loss has been reported in a few cases.

Voice Disorders: No voice disorders have been observed or reported.

Resonance Disorders: Hypernasal resonance may be present in cases with clefts.

Language Disorders: Severe language impairment is a constant feature of the syndrome.

Other Clinical Features:

Central nervous system: absence of the corpus callosum; arachnoid cysts; severe mental retardation; seizures; hypotonia; cortical atrophy;

Limbs and digits: preaxial polydactyly (dupication of the hallux); postaxial polydactyly; soft tissue syndactyly of two or more toes;

Craniofacial: macrocephaly; frontal bossing; prominent occiput; large anterior fontanel; hypertelorism; cleft lip and palate; depressed nasal root; strabismus; posteriorly rotated ears;

Cardiac: congenital heart anomalies;

Genitals: hypospadias; cryptorchidism;

Growth: short stature;

Abdominal: inguinal hernias; umbilical hernia.

Natural History: Growth deficiency is of postnatal onset and proportional. Neurologic and cognitive deficiency is apparent from infancy and initially presents as hypotonia. Seizures may also be apparent from infancy.

Treatment Prognosis: Depending on the severity of the central nervous system malformation, the prognosis for cognitive and language development is poor, as is the prognosis for normal speech development.

Differential Diagnosis: Hypertelorism, genital abnormalities, and clefting are common features of

Opitz syndrome which does not have as severe a developmental impairment. Clefting and polydactyly occur in several of the oral-facial-digital syndromes, some of which also have severe developmental impairment as a feature. Craniofacial anomalies, developmental impairment, and polydactyly are also found in **Carpenter syndrome.**

Acrodysostosis

Also Known As:

Acrodysostosis has often been lumped together with a number of other similar disorders that had a similar pattern of progression and anomalies, including Albright osteodystrophy and pseudohypoparathyroidism. However, acrodysostosis probably represents a separate and distinct disorder.

Major System(s) Affected:

Craniofacial; limbs; central nervous system; skeletal; growth.

Etiology: Autosomal dominant inheritance. The gene has not been identified or mapped.

Speech Disorders: Anterior skeletal open-bite or significant anterior cross-bite typically results in lingual protrusion during speech resulting in obligatory interdental distortions and substitutions. Because mental retardation is a common feature of this syndrome, some children with acrodysostosis have more severely impaired speech based on expressive language impairment.

Feeding Disorders: There are no specific feeding disorders known to be associated with acrodysostosis.

Hearing Disorders: There are no specific hearing disorders known to be associated with acrodysostosis.

Voice Disorders: There are no specific voice disorders known to be associated with acrodysostosis.

Resonance Disorders: There are no specific resonance disorders known to be associated with acrodysostosis.

Language Disorders: Language impairment is a common feature of the syndrome, with cognitive deficiency and developmental delay a component in a large majority of cases.

Other Clinical Features:

Craniofacial: maxillary deficiency with relative prognathism; small, short nose with anteverted nostrils;

Limbs: small hands and feet; cone-shaped epiphyses; abnormal metacarpals;

Central nervous system: cognitive impairment;

Musculoskeletal: advanced skeletal age with early ossification of bones;

Growth: short stature.

Natural History: Developmental delay is recognized early, but the impairment is static and nonprogressive. Birth weight and length are normal with growth deficiency becoming evident late in childhood.

Treatment Prognosis: Because the neurologic (cognitive) impairment is static, treatment for speech and language is indicated, though normal development should not be anticipated.

Differential Diagnosis: Acrodysostosis has been considered to overlap the disorders of Albright osteodystrophy and pseudohypoparathyroidism. However, acrodysostosis is now thought to be a distinct and separate disorder.

AEC Syndrome

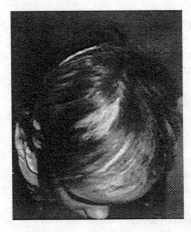

AEC syndrome: Note the sparse scalp hair associated with this form of ectodermal dysplasia.

Also Known As: Hay-Wells syndrome; ankyloblepheron-ecto-dermal defects-cleft lip/palate

AEC syndrome is one of several multiple anomaly syndromes that involve clefting of the lip and/or palate and ectodermal dysplasia. It is not known if there is a genotypic similarity between AEC syndrome and **Rapp-Hodgkin ectodermal dysplasia,** but there is substantial phenotypic overlap between these two disorders. AEC syndrome is one of a number of syndromes that may have cleft lip and palate as a feature, or cleft palate only (including submucous cleft) as a feature. It should be pointed out that if two

first-degree relatives have different cleft types (i.e., one has cleft palate only while the other has cleft lip and palate), this mixing of cleft types is a clear indication that the clefts are part of a syndrome.

Major System(s) Affected: Skin; nails; dental; integument; craniofacial.

Etiology: Autosomal dominant inheritance. The gene has not yet been identified or mapped.

Speech Disorders: Articulation disorders include obligatory distortions and substitutions secondary to small or missing teeth and cleft anomalies of the lip and dental alveolus. Compensatory articulation patterns secondary to clefting may also occur.

Feeding Disorders: There are no specific feeding problems except early difficulties related to clefting.

Hearing Disorders: Conductive hearing loss secondary to middle ear effusion is common.

Voice Disorders: Hoarseness is common, related to dryness of the vocal cords and the laryngeal mucosa.

Resonance Disorders: Hypernasality is common secondary to cleft palate.

Language Disorders: There is no language impairment associated with AEC syndrome.

Other Clinical Features:

Integument: ectodermal dysplasia; hypohidrosis; scalp lesions and infections; sparse hair of wiry texture; sparse or absent eyelashes; hypoplastic fingernails and toenails;

Dental: hypodontia;

Craniofacial: fusion of the eyelids by slender filiform adhesions; cleft lip with or without cleft palate; multiple alveolar frenula; maxillary hypoplasia.

Natural History: Ectodermal dysplasia is present from birth. Maxillary hypoplasia becomes progressively more severe with age and is in part related to alveolar bone degeneration related to hypodontia causing the mandible to over-rotate and making the chin more prominent.

Treatment Prognosis: With surgery and dental replacement, speech should be entirely normal, but therapy should be deferred until after physical management of the oral cavity is completed.

Differential Diagnosis: Syndromes with ectodermal dysplasia and clefting include **Rapp-Hodgkin syndrome** and **EEC syndrome** (Ectrodactyly-ectodermal dysplasia-clefting). It has been speculated that AEC syndrome is the same disorder as **Rapp-Hodgkin syndrome** with the exception of the filiform adhesions of the eyelids.

Aicardi Syndrome

Also Known As:

Aicardi syndrome is a rare disorder associated with cleft lip and palate that includes major anomalies of the central nervous system, including Dandy-Walker anomaly and lack of cerebral hemisphere differentiation (holoprosencephaly) in the most cases. The most severe expressions of this syndrome are incompatible with life.

Major System(s) Affected:
Central nervous system; craniofacial; ocular; vertebral; integument; limbs.

Etiology: X-linked dominant mapped to Xp22, lethal in males.

Speech Disorders: In many cases of Aicardi syndrome, the mental retardation is so severe that speech and language do not develop. However, in mildest cases, intellectual development can be relatively normal with essentially normal language development. Speech may be impaired by the effects of cleft lip and palate which is common in the syndrome.

Feeding Disorders: The severe central nervous system impairment in Aicardi syndrome may result in irritability and failure-to-thrive. Seizure activity may also interfere with feeding.

Hearing Disorders: No specific hearing impairments have been reported in Aicardi syndrome, although it is probable that patients with clefts may have an increased frequency of middle ear effusions and subsequent conductive hearing loss.

Voice Disorders: There are no known specific voice disorders.

Resonance Disorders: In cases with cleft lip and palate who develop language, hypernasal resonance secondary to the cleft is possible.

Language Disorders: Language impairment is present in nearly all cases, and in the most severely affected patients who survive the neonatal period, severe or absent language delay is likely.

Other Clinical Features:

Central nervous system: agenesis of the corpus callosum; heterotopia of the brain; mental retardation; flexion spasms in infancy; EEG abnormalities; seizures;

Craniofacial: cleft lip and palate;

Ocular: chorioretinal lacunae;

Skeletal: vertebral anomalies; scoliosis; rib anomalies;

Integument: lipomas on the scalp; cavernous hemangiomas.

Natural History: A significant percentage of neonates with Aicardi syndrome die in the neonatal period. Of those who survive, many have severe developmental impairment compounded by seizures and contractile spasms. The mildest cases, however, have had only minor cognitive impairments, but have had seizures and abnormal EEG patterns.

Treatment Prognosis: In the most severe cases, the prognosis for marked improvement in speech, language, and cognitive functioning is poor. Because cleft lip and palate are often present, clinicians may be misled into believing that the lack of speech development or early feeding difficulties are related to the cleft. However, in Aicardi syndrome, speech and feeding disorders are most likely to be caused by severe central nervous system impairment.

Differential Diagnosis: Absence of the corpus callosum in association with cleft lip and palate is common in **craniofrontonasal dysplasia.** Anomalies of the retina, specifically retinal coloboma, with clefting and central nervous system abnormalities is found in **holoprosencephaly, Kallmann syndrome,** and Roberts syndrome. Dandy-Walker anomaly and contractions are found in **Aase-Smith syndrome.**

Alagille Syndrome

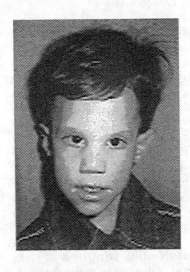

Alagille syndrome: Note the broad forehead, broad nasal root, and deep-set eyes associated with this syndrome.

Also Known As: Alagille-Watson syndrome, cholestasis with peripheral pulmonary stenosis, arteriohepatic dysplasia

Since 1975 Alagille syndrome has been recognized as a distinct syndrome with the association of a characteristic facial appearance with liver abnormalities and cognitive impairment. This rare disorder has a population frequency of approximately 1:70,000. Approximately 25% of individuals with Alagille syndrome do not survive past early childhood because of their cardiac or liver anomalies.

Major System(s) Affected: Craniofacial; ocular; cardiac; gastrointestinal; genitourinary; integument; skeletal; central nervous system; limbs.

Etiology: Autosomal dominant inheritance; mapped to 20p12 and may be caused by a contiguous gene deletion from 20p12.1-p11.23.

Speech Disorders: Speech may be delayed in some patients with Alagille syndrome, but acoustic production is generally normal.

Feeding Disorders: Early failure-to-thrive is common in patients with Alagille syndrome and has multifactorial causation. Intrahepatic duct anomalies, congenital heart anomalies, peripheral pulmonary stenosis, and mild hypotonia may all contribute to disinterest in feeding and poor weight gain in infancy.

Hearing Disorders: Hearing is generally within normal limits in Alagille syndrome.

Voice Disorders: Voice disorders have not been reported or observed in Alagille syndrome.

Resonance Disorders: Resonance disorders are not a component of Alagille syndrome.

Language Disorders: Language is delayed or mildly disordered in over 50% of patients with Alagille syndrome, but the disorders are not typically severe and may be at the outer limits of normal.

Other Clinical Features:

Craniofacial: broad forehead; pointed chin; prominent bulbous nasal tip; deep-set eyes;

Ocular: posterior embryotoxin, anterior chamber anomalies;

Cardiac: ventriculoseptal defect; atrial septal defect; pulmonic stenosis;

Gastrointestinal: liver anomalies and chronic liver disease (cholestasis) secondary to intrahepatic duct stenosis; newborn jaundice;

Genitourinary: kidney anomalies;

Integument: sparse facial and body hair in males;

Skeletal: vertebral anomalies; osteopenia; rib anomalies;

Central nervous system: mild cognitive impairment;

Limbs: short distal phalanges on both hands; short ulnas bilaterally.

Natural History: Liver disease is typically evident within the first few months of life so that failure-to-thrive typically presents early. Developmental milestones are usually slightly delayed. Quality and quantity of life is dependent on the cardiac anomalies and liver disease.

Treatment Prognosis: Feeding problems can be alleviated by medical treatment and are not related to mechanical factors. Other features of the syndrome can, in large part, be medically managed in many cases.

Differential Diagnosis: The combination of craniofacial abnormalities including deep-set eyes and pointed chin in association with peripheral pulmonary stenosis in **Williams syndrome.** However, Alagille syndrome may be differentiated by the presence of liver disease. The cognitive disorders are usually more significant in **Williams syndrome.**

Albers-Schönberg Syndrome

Also Known As: Osteopetrosis, autosomal recessive type; marble bones, autosomal recessive type; Albers-Schönberg disease

Albers-Schönberg syndrome is a severe, progressive bony overgrowth syndrome which has a poor long-term prognosis. Speech and hearing disorders progress as secondary manifestations of bony growth which impinges on the cranial nerves and mastoid bone.

Major System(s) Affected: Skeletal; craniofacial; central nervous system; ocular; dental; hematologic.

Etiology: Autosomal recessive inheritance. The gene has been mapped to 11q12-13.

Speech Disorders: There is progressive compression of multiple cranial nerves, including VII and VIII, which can lead to paresis of facial animation and movement resulting in articulatory distortions and oral resonance abnormalities. Delayed dental eruption may cause articulatory distortion. Hearing loss may also be progressive and

cause abnormalities of speech production. Osteomyelitis of the jaws may also cause restricted movement.

Feeding Disorders: If expressed early (congenital), failure-to-thrive may occur related to airway obstruction or cranial nerve abnormalities.

Hearing Disorders: There is progressive mixed or sensorineural hearing loss related to auditory nerve compression and progressive osteopetrosis which alters the ossicles and temporal bone.

Voice Disorders: Early voice production is normal. Hoarseness may develop in late childhood.

Resonance Disorders: Early resonance is normal, but hyponasality may develop in childhood or adolescence.

Language Disorders: A small percentage of individuals with Albers-Schönberg syndrome have cognitive impairment and may have language delay or disorder. However, the majority develop normal language before significant progression of the disease.

Other Clinical Features:

Skeletal: osteosclerosis; osteomyelitis;

Craniofacial: macrocephaly;

Central nervous system: hydrocephalus;

Ocular: progressive visual impairment from compression of the optic nerve; strabismus; nystagmus;

Dental: delayed dental eruption; rampant dental caries;

Hematologic: severe anemia; thrombocytopenia; pancytopenia;

Other: hepatosplenomegaly; early death (usually in second or third decade of life).

Natural History: The bony changes and anemia are progressive, creating a worsening of all symptoms and early death.

Treatment Prognosis: Long-term prognosis is poor.

Differential Diagnosis: There are many progressive bone disorders, including the craniotubular disorders (**craniometaphyseal dysplasia, frontometaphyseal dysplasia, craniodiaphyseal dysplasia, van Buchem syndrome, and** sclerosteosis), that have similar progressive features and comparable deterioration and symptoms. The blood disorders will help to differentiate Albers-Schönberg syndrome.

Angelman Syndrome

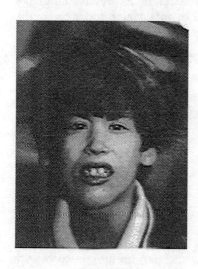

Angelman syndrome.

Also Known As: Happy puppet syndrome (*Note:* although this term has been applied in the past, it has a pejorative connotation in its attempt at humor and should be avoided as a diagnostic label)

Angelman syndrome is caused by the same chromosome deletion as **Prader-Willi syndrome,** but only when the deleted portion of the long arm of chromosome 15 is from the maternal chromosome. Absence of the maternal 15q11-q13 segment also causes Angelman syndrome if the affected individual has two 15q11-q13 segments, both from the father's chromosome 15 (paternal uniparental disomy). Alternately, **Prader-Willi syndrome** is caused by deletion of the paternal 15q11-q13. This expression of two different disorders based on the parental chromosome of origin is known as *imprinting.* There is essentially no phenotypic overlap between Angelman and **Prader-Willi syndromes.** Individuals with **Prader-Willi syndrome** do develop speech and language, whereas individuals with Angelman syndrome do not.

Major System(s) Affected:
Central nervous system; craniofacial; integument; dental.

Etiology: Deletion of 15q11-q13 from the maternal chromosome 15 (imprinting) or lack of maternal 15q11-q13 caused by uniparental disomy.

Speech Disorders: There is no speech development in individuals with Angelman syndrome.

Feeding Disorders: There may be early failure-to-thrive related to severe hypotonia and later in life, feeding is complicated by persistent protrusion of the tongue and severe ataxia.

Hearing Disorders: Hearing is usually within normal limits.

Voice Disorders: Speech does not develop in this syndrome and voice is therefore limited to random noises and grunts.

Resonance Disorders: Resonance is not an issue because of the lack of speech development.

Language Disorders: Although there is minimal receptive language development in some cases, the majority of individuals with Angelman syndrome are severely retarded and have progressive ataxia. Expressive language does not develop and is one of the hallmarks of the syndrome.

Other Clinical Features:

Central nervous system: progressive ataxia; hyperactive reflexes; hypotonia in infancy; wild outbursts of laughter; cortical atrophy; seizures; abnormal EEG patterns; arm flapping;

Craniofacial: relative prognathism secondary to a long mandibular body and maxillary deficiency; persistent open-mouth posture with tongue protrusion; macrostomia; microcephaly; brachycephaly;

Integument: anomalous pigmentation of the choroid; hypopigmented areas of skin;

Dental: dental spacing.

Natural History: Birth weight and head circumference at birth are normal, but abnormal psychomotor development is immediately obvious and hypotonia is evident at birth. With age, ataxia and involuntary movements develop and become progressively worse, accompanied by seizures. There is persistent protrusive posturing of the tongue with paroxysmal laughter and arm flapping.

Treatment Prognosis: Poor.

Differential Diagnosis: The profile of ataxia and behavior patterns seen in Angelman syndrome are distinctive. However, progressive ataxia and skin pigmentation anomalies are also seen in **ataxia-telangiectasia syndrome.** However, cognition is not as severely impaired in **ataxia-telangiectasia syndrome.**

Antley-Bixler Syndrome

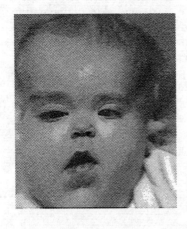

Antley-Bixler syndrome: Note the abnormal head shape, depressed nasal root, and ear abnormality.

Also Known As: ABS; trapezoidocephaly-synostosis syndrome; multisynostotic osteodysgenesis

Antley-Bixler syndrome is a rare syndrome of craniosynostosis that has many extracranial anomalies primarily involving the limbs and joints. The craniofacial anomalies are very severe and many infants with Antley-Bixler syndrome die in infancy from airway complications.

Major System(s) Affected: Craniofacial; limbs; skeletal; genitourinary.

Etiology: Autosomal recessive inheritance. The gene has not yet been identified or mapped.

Speech Disorders: Articulation is impaired by severe maxillary deficiency, Class III malocclusion, skeletal open-bite resulting in persistent tongue protrusion, severe restriction of oral cavity size, and nasal obstruction.

Feeding Disorders: Early feeding is impaired by respiratory compromise and nasal obstruction. Neonates with Antley-Bixler syndrome cannot breathe and eat simultaneously and their respiratory compromise must be dealt with prior to resolving their feeding problems.

Hearing Disorders: Conductive hearing loss is undoubtedly common in the syndrome, although there have been no specific reports describing hearing.

Voice Disorders: None have been reported or observed.

Resonance Disorders: Hyponasality is common secondary to nasal obstruction, choanal atresia, or a small nasal capsule.

Language Disorders: Expressive language may be impaired, but there are patients with Antley-Bixler syndrome who have had normal cognition and intellectual development.

Other Clinical Features:

Craniofacial: severe maxillary deficiency; depressed nasal root; frontal bossing; exorbitism; choanal stenosis or atresia;

Limb: joint contractures of the elbows, knees, and digits; radiohumeral synostosis; femoral bowing; femoral fractures; ulnar bowing; rocker-bottom feet;

Skeletal: rib anomalies; narrow iliac wings; hip dislocations;

Genitourinary: urinary tract anomalies in females and imperforate anus have been observed.

Natural History: The various synostoses in Antley-Bixler syndrome are progressive and the craniofacial anomalies may become significantly more pronounced with age. Early death from airway obstruction occurs in a high percentage of patients with this syndrome, so aggressive treatment for airway obstruction, including tracheotomy, is indicated.

Treatment Prognosis: With early correction of airway obstruction, and eventual craniofacial surgery, there is the possibility that individuals with Antley-Bixler syndrome can develop normal cognition, speech, and language. However, many speech disorders are obligatory in nature and cannot be resolved with reconstructive surgery for craniofacial anomalies.

Differential Diagnosis: Several syndromes of craniosynostosis have unusual limb anomalies. **Baller-Gerold syndrome** has absence or hypoplasia of the radius and digital anomalies, but the craniofacial anomalies are not similar to those seen in Antley-Bixler syndrome. Craniosynostosis may accompany other syndromes with contractures, including arthrogryposis. Multiple synostosis syndrome may have similar limb anomalies in association with minor craniofacial anomalies. **Pfeiffer syndrome** has similar craniofacial anomalies with minor anomalies of the digits.

Apert Syndrome

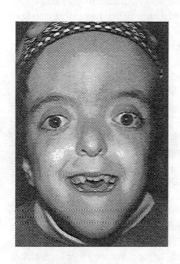

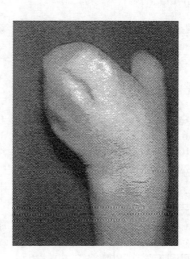

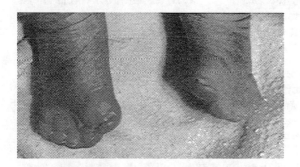

Apert syndrome: Note the orbital hypertelorism and anterior skeletal open-bite and syndactyly of the hands and feet.

31

Also Known As: Acrocephalosyndactyly

Major System(s) Affected: Craniofacial; limb; central nervous system; growth.

Etiology: Single gene, autosomal dominantly inherited disorder caused by a mutation in the FGFR2 gene (fibroblast growth factor receptor 2) located on the long arm of chromosome 10.

Speech Disorders: Articulation impairment related to malocclusion and open-bite with obligatory tongue placement errors resulting in anterior articulatory distortions. Because the maxilla is hypoplastic, the tongue often remains in the floor of the mouth with little or no articulatory placement in the maxillary arch.

Feeding Disorders: Upper airway obstruction and possible choanal atresia will result in failure-to-thrive because infants with Apert syndrome will strive to maintain respiration even at the expense of feeding. In such cases, the airway obstruction must be relieved.

Hearing Disorders: Conductive hearing loss, usually mild to moderate, is common and may be related to chronic middle ear disease, chronic fluid, ossicular anomalies, or any combination of the three.

Voice Disorders: Hoarseness is occasionally present in childhood and adolescence and may be related to premature ossification of the thyroid, cricoid, or tracheal cartilages.

Resonance Disorders: Hyponasality is very common and may be related to choanal atresia or stenosis, or to the small nasopharynx. In cases where cleft palate is found, mixed hyper/hyponasality may be present, but hyponasality is far more common.

Language Disorders: Language delay is common and may then develop with specific disorders related to cognitive deficiency. However, most children with Apert syndrome do develop adequate receptive and expressive language skills for communication. In the most severely affected cases, expressive language does not develop.

Other Clinical Features:

  Craniofacial: synostosis of multiple cranial and facial

sutures; maxillary hypoplasia; class III malocclusion; open-bite; cleft palate; choanal atresia or stenosis; small nasal cavity; orbital hypertelorism; low set posteriorly rotated ears; synostosis (fusion) of one or more ossicles; fixation of the footplate of the stapes; reduced size of middle ear space; chronic serous otitis; Eustachian tube dysfunction may be caused by abnormal angulation of the Eustachian tube orifice and reduced diameter of the tube because of abnormal bone growth of the surrounding craniofacial skeleton;

Limbs: syndactyly of fingers and toes; brachymelia (short forearms); acne vulgaris;

Central nervous system: mental retardation, macrencephaly, hydrocephalus, increased intracranial pressure;

Growth: occasional short stature.

Natural History: Newborns with Apert syndrome have variable expression of the craniofacial findings, but fusion of all of the digits on all limbs occurs in most cases.

Choanal atresia or stenosis results in early airway obstruction and possible severe obstructive apnea, which may require emergency treatment, including possible tracheotomy. Craniofacial findings progress following birth and abnormal craniofacial growth becomes evident early in life, usually before 2 years of age. In some cases, craniofacial findings are severe at birth. Developmental delay is common, although some patients have normal cognition and development. In some cases, however, cognitive impairment is severe. Class III malocclusion with developing open-bite is often evident by school age. Craniosynostosis continues after birth resulting in progressive distortion of the cranial bones and progressive midface hypoplasia. Learning disorders are usually evident early in life and mental retardation or learning disabilities often result in special class placement. The majority of children with Apert syndrome have some type of cognitive impairment. Life expectancy is normal.

Treatment Prognosis: Articulation disorders associated with Apert syndrome in childhood would be resistant to speech therapy because of the structural anomalies of the oral cavity. The errors are obligatory and would not be expected to resolve without surgical reconstruction of the craniofacial skeleton with craniofacial and/or orthognathic procedures. Language impairment will often respond to treatment, but progress may be limited by cognitive impairment. Hyponasality is also obligatory and can only be resolved with surgical management of the midface hypoplasia. Choanal stenosis or atresia are typically resistant to surgical resolution because of progressive skeletal dysplasia and because children with Apert syndrome are chronic mouth breathers. Lack of nasal respiration will prevent the nasal cavity from remaining patent, even after surgical repair. Hearing loss will also necessitate surgical resolution.

Differential Diagnosis: There are several other syndromes which have the association of craniosynostosis and limb anomalies including **Saethre-Chotzen syndrome, Pfeiffer syndrome, Jackson-Weiss syndrome,** and **Shprintzen-Goldberg syndrome.** Although the craniofacial anomalies in these syndromes are similar to those seen in Apert syndrome, only children with Apert syndrome have the "mitten hand" resulting from the syndactyly of all of the fingers or fusion of all of the toes. **Crouzon syndrome** has similar craniofacial anomalies, but no syndactyly. Interestingly, **Jackson-Weiss** and **Crouzon syndrome** are caused by a different mutation in the same FGFR2 gene as Apert syndrome.

Ascher Syndrome

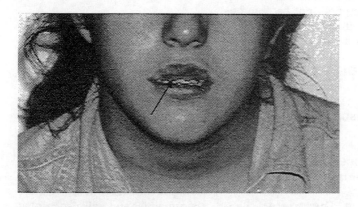

Ascher syndrome: Note the extra fold of skin, often described as a "double lip" (arrow).

Also Known As: Blepharochalasis and double lip

Ascher syndrome was first described early in the 20th century, and a substantial number of cases of this rare syndrome have been described since, largely because the facial manifestations are so distinctive. The upper eyelids droop, often narrowing the palpebral fissures, and there is a second fold of liplike tissue running parallel and under the upper lip. Individuals with this dominantly inherited syndrome are developmentally normal.

Major System(s) Affected: Facial; endocrine.

Etiology: Autosomal dominant inheritance. The gene has not been identified or mapped as yet.

Speech Disorders: The redundancy of lip tissue can cause minor distortions of some sounds, including bilabials, but other anterior sounds can be altered by the redundancy of lip tissue which will constrict the oral opening. These distortions are obligatory in nature.

Feeding Disorders: No feeding disorders have been noted. The lip redundancy does not become noticeable until after infancy, usually in childhood.

Hearing Disorders: Hearing is normal.

Voice Disorders: Voice is normal.

Resonance Disorders: Resonance is normal.

Language Disorders: Language development is normal.

Other Clinical Features:

> **Facial:** blepharochalasis (drooping upper eyelids); duplication of the upper lip and occasioanl edema of the lower lip;
>
> **Endocrine:** benign enlargement of the thyroid gland

which is only occasionally symptomatic.

Natural History: The lip and eyelid anomalies are not apparent at birth. The lip duplication becomes apparent in childhood and the blepharochalasis becomes obvious by puberty. The thyroid enlargement is the last of the clinical features to be expressed.

Treatment Prognosis: Surgical reconstruction of both the eyelid and lip anomalies can resolve these abnormalities and will also resolve the speech distortions.

Differential Diagnosis: Redundancy of facial soft tissues, including the upper lip and eyelids is a feature of **Setleis syndrome**. However, the soft tissue redundancy in **Setleis syndrome** is more generalized to all of the facial soft tissues.

Ataxia-telangiectasia Syndrome

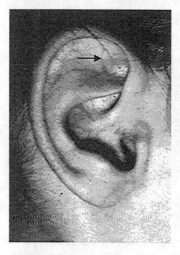

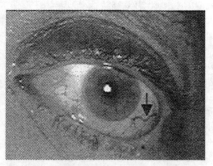

Ataxia-telangiectasia syndrome: Note the telangiectasias in the ear and eye (arrows).

Also Known As: Louis-Bar syndrome

Ataxia-telangiectasia syndrome is a progressive degenerative neurological disorder usually resulting in early death, usually by 20 years of age. It has a population prevalence of approximately 1:100,000, although some believe this to be an underestimate. Gene carriers of this recessive disorder are probably fairly common. The syndrome is a particularly devastating one because early development is normal with degeneration beginning in childhood. As an autosomal recessive disorder, a high percentage of cases come as a surprise to parents because the disorder may not have previously been seen in the family.

Major System(s) Affected: Central nervous system; integument.

Etiology: Autosomal recessive mutation, mapped to 11q22.3.

Speech Disorders: Ataxia-telangiectasia is a progressive disorder with onset in early childhood,

37

usually by 3 years of age. Early motor development is normal, including speech onset. Cerebellar ataxia becomes apparent in childhood followed by dystonia. Speech becomes progressively more dysarthric and often becomes unintelligible.

Feeding Disorders: Early feeding is normal, but after the onset of ataxia, there is often copious drooling and poor oral-motor control. However, oral feeding is preserved, although the ability to orally manipulate food and masticate is impaired.

Hearing Disorders: There are no known hearing impairments in ataxia-telangiectasia syndrome.

Voice Disorders: Voice becomes tremulous and weak after the onset of ataxia and becomes progressively worse with age.

Resonance Disorders: Hypernasality is often present after the onset and progression of ataxia.

Language Disorders: Early language development is normal, and cognition is also normal in childhood, although there is a plateau of cognitive development in late childhood. However, receptive language remains intact.

Other Clinical Features:

> **Central nervous system:** progressive ataxia; tremors;
>
> **Integument:** telangiectasias;
>
> **Other:** development of neoplasias.

Natural History: The face becomes thin, drawn, and expressionless. Upper extremity tremors are common. Telangiectasias begin to become apparent in childhood after the onset of ataxia, but are not present in all patients. There are recurrent upper and lower respiratory infections with immune deficiency present in most cases. There is a high frequency of malignant neoplasia development, including leukemia and both Hodgkin's disease and non-Hodgkin lymphoma. Life span is shortened with death often occurring before 20 years of age from cancer or severe respiratory disorders. Some patients, however, have lived into their 40s. The disorder is progressive.

Treatment Prognosis: Because of the progressive nature of the disorder, there are no known effective treatments for the ataxia or speech and feeding disorders. Because there is a DNA repair defect associated with the syndrome, some conventional therapies for cancers are also ineffective or may even exacerbate the problem.

Differential Diagnosis: There are other progressive neurologic disorders which also involve skin changes, including Refsum syndrome and a number of other genetic (usually recessive) conditions which involve progressive ataxia. However, many of these syndromes also involve hearing loss and the skin changes are more closely related to ichthyosis than telangiectasia.

Baller-Gerold Syndrome

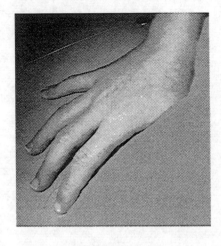

Absence of the thumb in Baller-Gerold syndrome.

Also Known As: BGS, craniosynostosis-radial aplasia syndrome

Baller-Gerold syndrome is a rare disorder with striking limb anomalies as the most distinctive features. Although craniosynostosis is also a clinical finding, it is not the same type of pansynostosis typically seen in **Crouzon** or **Apert syndromes** and the skull malformations are usually not as severe. Cleft palate is an occasional finding.

Major System(s) Affected: Craniofacial; limb; central nervous system; growth; skeletal; intestinal; genitourinary; cardiac.

Etiology: Autosomal recessive inheritance. The gene has not been identified or mapped as yet.

Speech Disorders: Articulation disorders are found on occasion. In some instances, articulation impairment is secondary to cleft palate and velopharyngeal insufficiency. In other cases, there are obligatory placement errors related to micrognathia and Class II malocclusion.

Feeding Disorders: Neonatal failure-to-thrive may occur secondary to brain anomalies and/or cardiac malformations. However, swallowing is not specifically impaired.

Hearing Disorders: Conductive hearing loss is a common feature.

Voice Disorders: Voice is normal.

Resonance Disorders: Hypernasal resonance may occur in cases with cleft palate. However, hyponasality is not a prominent feature of this syndrome as it is in other syndromes of craniosynostosis.

Language Disorders: Language is impaired in cases with neurologic impairment and developmental delay.

Other Clinical Features:

Craniofacial: craniosynostosis; micrognathia; posteriorly sloping forehead; prominent nasal root; epicanthal folds; small posteriorly rotated ears;

Limb and skeletal: absent radius; anomalous ulna; carpal and metacarpal aplasia; absent or hypoplastic thumbs; vertebral anomalies; rib anomalies;

Central nervous system: polymicrogyria; cognitive impairment;

Growth: short stature;

Intestinal: imperforate or anteriorly displaced anus; rectovaginal fistula;

Genitourinary: crossed renal ectopia;

Cardiac: ventriculoseptal defect; patent ductus arteriosus

Natural History: The disorder is a static one, but there have been reports of infant deaths related to brain anomalies in a small number of cases. Most cases survive and a percentage have normal intellect and cognitive development.

Treatment Prognosis: The prognosis for normal speech is good if cognitive impairment is not too severe. Craniofacial surgery can correct the cranial and jaw anomalies. The limb malformations, depending on severity, may not be completely resolved, but appropriate surgical and motor compensations can be made.

Differential Diagnosis: Limb and craniofacial anomalies involving limb reduction may be found in Holt-Oram syndrome and **Antley-Bixler syndrome.** Radial anomalies with absent thumbs and micrognathia is found in **Nager syndrome.**

Bamatter Syndrome

Also Known As: Geroderma osteodysplastica, Walt Disney dwarfing (*Note:* although this term has been applied in the past, it has a pejorative connotation by equating the appearance of affected individuals with the characters from Disney's *Snow White* and should therefore be avoided as a diagnostic label).

This syndrome of short stature is rare, but distinctive in its phenotype. The short stature is often mildly disproportionate with the trunk being more severely affected than the limbs, which may therefore seem disproportionately long. Performance and intellect are normal. The most noticeable facial manifestation is skin laxity which gives the face a prematurely aged appearance. The bones are fragile and prone to fracture.

Major System(s) Affected: Growth; integument; musculoskeletal; craniofacial.

Etiology: Autosomal recessive inheritance. The gene has not been identified or mapped as yet.

Speech Disorders: Articulatory distortions secondary to malocclusion is common. Mandibular prognathism is a common feature caused in part by decreased alveolar bone height resulting in overclosure of the mandible. The malocclusion may distort anterior sounds, especially lingua-alveolar sounds.

Feeding Disorders: Feeding is not known to be impaired in Bamatter syndrome.

Hearing Disorders: Hearing is not known to be impaired in Bamatter syndrome.

Voice Disorders: Voice is usually high pitched and may be hoarse, related to premature ossification of the larynx.

Resonance Disorders: Resonance is not impaired in Bamatter syndrome.

Language Disorders: Language development is normal.

Other Clinical Features:

   Growth: short stature;

Integument: lax facial skin;

Musculoskeletal: osteoporosis; susceptibility to bone fractures; abnormal vertebrae; scoliosis and/or lordosis; hypotonia; pectus carinatum; joint laxity; hip dislocation;

Craniofacial: relative mandibular prognathism; depressed malar eminences.

Natural History: Growth deficiency is postnatal, but the syndrome's joint and skin laxity become apparent very early. The skeletal dysplasia is progressive.

Treatment Prognosis: The articulation disorders related to the prognathism are difficult to treat. Osteotomies of the jaw to correct the prognathism are problematic because of the tendency for the bones to fracture and splinter. The articulatory distortions are obligatory in nature, and therefore, will probably persist without correction of the structural anomaly.

Differential Diagnosis: Skin laxity is common in a number of disorders, including Ehlers-Danlos syndrome, **Setleis syndrome,** and acrogeria. A prematurely aged facies without cognitive impairment is seen in progeria and granddad syndrome.

Bannayan-Zonana Syndrome

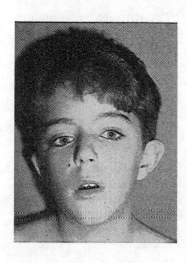

Macrocephaly and mild hypertelorism in Bannayan-Zonana syndrome.

Also Known As: Bannayan-Riley-Ruvalcaba syndrome; Riley-Smith syndrome; Ruvalcaba-Myrhe syndrome; Ruvalcaba-Myrhe-Smith syndrome

Initially described in 1971, the frequency of this disorder is unknown and is probably underestimated because of a lack of major dysmorphic findings. Neonates with this syndrome are large, often over 4 kg (9 pounds). However, growth is not accelerated after birth, and other than macrencephaly, individuals with Bannayan-Zonana syndrome are not abnormally large. Cognitive impairment, ranging from mild to severe, is found in over half of patients. Over 80% of reported cases have been male, but some of the male predominance may be related to the diagnostic significance of male genital abnormalities.

Major System(s) Affected: Craniofacial; skin; central nervous system; ocular; limbs; muscles; endocrine; genitals.

Etiology: Autosomal dominant mode of inheritance. The gene, labelled as PTEN, has been mapped to 10q23.3.

Speech Disorders: Speech is typically delayed and mild dysarthria occurs in some cases. Articulation impairment related to a global speech delay is common.

Feeding Disorders: Drooling has been noted in some patients. Early feeding may be difficult because of hypotonia, but failure-to-thrive has not been a major problem.

Hearing Disorders: Hearing impairment has not been reported in Bannayan-Zonana syndrome.

Voice Disorders: Voice disorders are not a feature of Bannayan-Zonana syndrome.

Resonance Disorders: Hypernasality has been observed in some patients as a component of a mildly dysarthric speech pattern. Velopharyngeal insufficiency skewed to one side of the pharynx may be caused by asymmetric movement of the velum and/or lateral pharyngeal walls.

Language Disorders: Language has been delayed and impaired in over half of observed cases.

Other Clinical Features:

Growth: high birth weight;

Craniofacial: macrocephaly; scaphocephaly; delayed closure of the anterior fontanelle; mild hypertelorism;

Skin: hemangiomas; lipomas; telengiectasias; cutis marmorata; café-au-lait spots;

Central nervous system: hypotonia; cognitive impairment, delay in motor milestones; macrencephaly; susceptibility to intracranial tumors;

Ocular: strabismus (exotropia); pseudopapilledema;

Limbs: broad thumbs and halluces;

Muscles: myopathy;

Endocrine: thyroid disease or thyroid tumors;

Genitals: macropenis; enlarged testes; dark spots on the glans of the penis.

Natural History: The myopathic process and the development of neoplasias is a progressive condition, but the developmental delay and cognitive impairment are static.

Treatment Prognosis: The outcome for the resolution of speech and language impairment is dependent on the degree of central nervous system involvement and cognitive deficiency. Some patients have fairly normal cognition, but at the other end of the spectrum, some patients are severely retarded. The dysarthria and articulation impairment seen in Bannayan-Zonana syndrome may improve with speech therapy, but complete normalization should not be expected in severe cases.

Differential Diagnosis: Macrencephaly with café-au-lait spots are features of neurofibromatosis type I. Peutz-Jerger syndrome has similar genital pigmentation anomalies, although the pigmented maculae are seen on other parts of the body as well.

Bardet-Biedl Syndrome, Type 1

Also Known As: BBS1

Prior to the application of molecular genetics techniques, the association of obesity, pigmentary retinopathy, and mental retardation was classified as Laurence-Moon-Bardet-Biedl syndrome. It is now known, however, that all of the cases initially lumped together under Lawrence-Moon-Bardet-Biedl syndrome do not represent the same disorder. Four subtypes of Bardet-Biedl syndrome and a single type of **Lawrence-Moon syndrome** have now become recognized as distinct syndromes with identifiable etiologies. All of these disorders have mental retardation as a constant finding.

Major System(s) Affected: Central nervous system; endocrine/growth; ocular; genitourinary; limbs.

Etiology: Autosomal recessive mode of inheritance. The gene has been mapped to 11q13.

Speech Disorders: Speech is typically very delayed and in the most severe cases, speech may be very limited. Severe hypotonia may further impair articulation development.

Feeding Disorders: Severe hypotonia may result in a weak suck in infancy.

Hearing Disorders: Hearing is not impaired.

Voice Disorders: Voice may be weak or breathy.

Resonance Disorders: Resonance is normal.

Language Disorders: Language is always impaired in Bardet-Biedl syndrome, type 1. There is always significant delay in the onset of language milestones, and language develops slowly.

Other Clinical Features:

Central nervous system: mental retardation; hypotonia;

Endocrine/growth: obesity;

Ocular: pigmentary retinopathy;

Genitourinary: micropenis; hypogonadism;

Limbs: polydactyly.

Natural History: The developmental impairment associated with Bardet-Biedl syndrome, type 1 is present from birth and remains static throughout life. The retinopathy is progressive with onset in childhood, usually after 5 years of age. Eventual blindness occurs in most patients by the third decade of life.

Treatment Prognosis: The overall prognosis for marked improvement in cognitive develop-

ment and language is poor. As visual impairment progresses, the cognitive impairments may be exacerbated.

B

Differential Diagnosis: There are other syndromes that have cognitive impairment, obesity, and hypotonia as features, including **Laurence-Moon syndrome, Prader-Willi syndrome** and **Cohen syndrome.** However, **Prader-Willi syndrome, Cohen syndrome,** and **Laurence-Moon syndrome** do not have polydactyly as a feature. **Laurence-Moon syndrome** also has spastic paraplegia as a feature, unlike Bardet-Biedl syndrome, type 1.

Bardet-Biedl Syndrome, Type 2

Also Known As: BBS2

Bardet-Biedl syndrome, type 2, differs from type 1 with the addition of hypertension, diabetes mellitus, and liver disease as clinical features. The syndrome has the same pattern of inheritance, but a different gene and gene locus are involved.

Major System(s) Affected: Central nervous system; endocrine/growth; ocular; genitourinary/renal; limbs; liver.

Etiology: Autosomal recessive mode of inheritance. The gene has been mapped to 16q21.

Speech Disorders: Speech is typically very delayed, and in the most severe cases, speech may be very limited. Severe hypotonia may further impair articulation development.

Feeding Disorders: Severe hypotonia may result in a weak suck in infancy.

Hearing Disorders: Hearing is not impaired.

Voice Disorders: Voice may be weak or breathy.

Resonance Disorders: Resonance is normal.

Language Disorders: Language is always impaired in Bardet-Biedl syndrome, type 2. There is always significant delay in the onset of language milestones, and language develops slowly.

Other Clinical Features:

Central nervous system: mental retardation; hypotonia;

Endocrine/growth: obesity; diabetes mellitus;

Ocular: pigmentary retinopathy;

Genitourinary/renal: micropenis; hypogonadism; kidney failure;

Limbs: polydactyly; syndactyly; brachydactyly;

Liver: hepatic fibrosis;

Other: hypertension.

Natural History: The developmental impairment associated with Bardet-Biedl, type 2, is present from birth and remains static throughout life. The retinopathy is progressive with onset in childhood, usually after 5 years of age. Eventual blindness occurs in most patients by the third decade of life.

Treatment Prognosis: The overall prognosis for marked improvement in cognitive development and language is poor. As visual impairment progresses, the cognitive impairments may be exacerbated.

Differential Diagnosis: There are other syndromes that have cognitive impairment, obesity, and hypotonia as features, including **Laurence-Moon syndrome,** Prader-Willi syndrome and **Cohen syndrome.** However, **Prader-Willi syndrome, Cohen syndrome,** and **Laurence-Moon syndrome** do not have polydactyly as a feature. **Laurence-Moon syndrome** also has spastic paraplegia as a feature, unlike Bardet-Biedl syndrome, type 2.

B

Bardet-Biedl Syndrome, Type 3

Also Known As: BBS3

Bardet-Biedl syndrome, type 3, is phenotypically very similar to Bardet-Biedl syndrome, type 2, including the presence of hypertension, diabetes mellitus, and liver disease as clinical features. The syndrome has the same pattern of inheritance, but a different gene and gene locus are involved.

Major System(s) Affected: Central nervous system; endocrine/growth; ocular; genitourinary/renal; limbs; liver.

Etiology: Autosomal recessive mode of inheritance. The gene has been mapped to 3p13-p12.

Speech Disorders: Speech is typically very delayed and, in the most severe cases, speech may be very limited. Severe hypotonia may further impair articulation development.

Feeding Disorders: Severe hypotonia may result in a weak suck in infancy.

Hearing Disorders: Hearing is not impaired.

Voice Disorders: Voice may be weak or breathy.

Resonance Disorders: Resonance is normal.

Language Disorders: Language is always impaired in Bardet-Biedl syndrome, type 3. There is always significant delay in the onset of language milestones, and language develops slowly.

Other Clinical Features:

Central nervous system: mental retardation; hypotonia;

Endocrine/growth: obesity; diabetes mellitus;

Ocular: pigmentary retinopathy;

Genitourinary/renal: micropenis; hypogonadism; kidney failure;

Limbs: polydactyly; syndactyly; brachydactyly;

Liver: hepatic fibrosis;

Other: hypertension.

Natural History: The developmental impairment associated with Bardet-Biedl, type 3, is present from birth and remains static throughout life. The retinopathy is progressive with onset in childhood, usually after 5 years of age. Eventual blindness occurs in most patients by the third decade of life.

Treatment Prognosis: The overall prognosis for marked improvement in cognitive development and language is poor. As visual impairment progresses, the cognitive impairments may be exacerbated.

Differential Diagnosis: There are other syndromes that have cognitive impairment, obesity, and hypotonia as features, including **Laurence-Moon syndrome, Prader-Willi syndrome,** and **Cohen syndrome.** However, **Prader-Willi syndrome, Cohen syndrome,** and **Laurence-Moon syndrome** do not have polydactyly as a feature. **Laurence-Moon syndrome** also has spastic paraplegia as a feature, unlike Bardet-Biedl syndrome, type 3.

Bardet-Biedl Syndrome, Type 4

Also Known As: BBS4

Bardet-Biedl syndrome, type 4, is phenotypically very similar to Bardet-Biedl syndrome, types 2 and 3, including the presence of hypertension, diabetes mellitus, and liver disease as clinical features. The syndrome has the same pattern of inheritance, but a different gene and gene locus are involved.

Major System(s) Affected: Central nervous system; endocrine/growth; ocular; genitourinary/renal; limbs; liver.

Etiology: Autosomal recessive mode of inheritance. The gene has been mapped to 15q22.3-q23.

Speech Disorders: Speech is typically very delayed and, in the most severe cases, speech may be very limited. Severe hypotonia may further impair articulation development.

Feeding Disorders: Severe hypotonia may result in a weak suck in infancy.

Hearing Disorders: Hearing is not impaired.

Voice Disorders: Voice may be weak or breathy.

Resonance Disorders: Resonance is normal.

Language Disorders: Language is always impaired in Bardet-Biedl syndrome, type 4. There is always significant delay in the onset of language milestones, and language develops slowly.

Other Clinical Features:

Central nervous system: mental retardation; hypotonia;

Endocrine/growth: obesity; diabetes mellitus;

Ocular: pigmentary retinopathy;

Genitourinary/renal: micropenis; hypogonadism; kidney failure;

Limbs: polydactyly; syndactyly; brachydactyly;

Liver: hepatic fibrosis;

Other: hypertension.

Natural History: The developmental impairment associated with Bardet-Biedl, type 4, is present from birth and remains static throughout life. The retinopathy is progressive with onset in childhood, usually after 5 years of age. Eventual blindness occurs in most patients by the third decade of life.

Treatment Prognosis: The overall prognosis for marked improvement in cognitive development and language is poor. As visual impairment progresses, the cognitive impairments may be exacerbated.

Differential Diagnosis: There are other syndromes that have cognitive impairment, obesity, and hypotonia as features, including **Laurence-Moon syndrome, Prader-Willi syndrome** and **Cohen syndrome.** However, **Prader-Willi syndrome, Cohen syndrome,** and **Laurence-Moon syndrome** do not have polydactyly as a feature. **Laurence-Moon syndrome** also has spastic paraplegia as a feature, unlike Bardet-Biedl syndrome, type 4.

Basal Cell Nevus Syndrome

Also Known As: Gorlin syndrome; Gorlin-Goltz syndrome

Basal cell nevus syndrome is relatively rare, occurring in less than 1:50,000 live births. However, the syndrome is common among individuals who have basal cell carcinomas (approximately 1:200). The carcinomas do not occur in all patients with the syndrome, but are found in most. The onset of the tumors is usually near or after the onset of puberty. Cognitive impairment is not a common feature of the syndrome, probably occurring in less than 5%. Nearly 50% of cases are new mutations.

Major System(s) Affected: Integument; craniofacial; central nervous system; ocular; musculoskeletal; limbs; gastrointestinal; genitourinary; cardiac; pulmonary.

Etiology: Autosomal dominant inheritance. A deletion has been mapped to 9q22.3.

Speech Disorders: Speech production may be adversely affected by clefting (an uncommon finding in the syndrome) or the late-onset development of jaw cysts. Speech is normal in most cases.

Feeding Disorders: Neonatal feeding disorders have not been reported or documented. Adult eating may be impacted by jaw cysts.

Hearing Disorders: Hearing is typically normal.

Voice Disorders: There have been no reports of voice disorders.

Resonance Disorders: Hypernasal resonance secondary to cleft palate may occur.

Language Disorders: Language is impaired in 10% or less of cases related to congenital brain malformations with cognitive deficiency.

Other Clinical Features:

Integument: basal cell nevi and/or carcinomas;

Craniofacial: prognathism; frontal bossing; macrocephaly; jaw cysts; round, broad face; hypertelorism; cleft lip and/or palate;

Central nervous system: cognitive deficiency; agenesis of the corpus callosum;

Ocular: strabismus; ocular dermoid cysts; iris coloboma; congenital cataract; glaucoma;

Musculoskeletal: rib anomalies; kyphoscoliosis; Sprengel shoulder;

Limbs: polydactyly; brachydactyly; pectus excavatum;

Gastrointestinal: gastrointestinal cysts and polyps;

Genitourinary: ovarian fibromas or carcinomas; male genital hypoplasia;

Cardiac: cardiac fibromas;

Pulmonary: lung cysts.

Natural History: The expression of the disorder is often not apparent until skin lesions become obvious in late childhood or adolescence. Neoplasias and/or hamartomas represent a progressive disorder.

Treatment Prognosis: Symptomatic treatment is usually successful, but careful examination for neoplasias is recommended.

Differential Diagnosis: There are many syndromes that have multiple skin lesions as a prominent feature, including **LEOPARD syndrome** and Peutz-Jerger syndrome. However, the distribution and location of nevi or skin pigment abnormalities are different. **LEOPARD syndrome** is usually accompanied by cognitive impairment and many individuals have hearing loss.

Beckwith-Wiedemann Syndrome

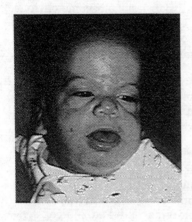

Prognathism and macroglossia in an infant with Beckwith-Wiedemann syndrome.

Also Known As: Wiedemann-Beckwith syndrome; exomphalos-macroglossia, gigantism syndrome (EMG syndrome)

Beckwith-Wiedemann syndrome is a relatively common multiple anomaly syndrome, and perhaps the most common overgrowth syndrome in humans, with a frequency of approximately 1:13,000 live births. Essentially, all children with Beckwith-Wiedemann syndrome have speech and language impairment, although it is typically mild. The syndrome is almost always detected initially in infancy because of abdominal abnormalities, metabolic disorders, or overgrowth coupled with hypotonia. It should be of particular interest to speech-language pathologists because of macroglossia and mandibular prognathism coupled with hypotonia, which causes a wide array of articulation disorders. Cleft palate, including a high prevalence of submucous cleft palate, may further complicate speech disorders.

Major System(s) Affected: Growth; craniofacial; gastrointestinal/abdominal; metabolic/endocrine; genital, motor development; central nervous system.

Etiology: Autosomal dominant inheritance. Several mechanisms

58

for the disorder have been reported, including a contiguous gene duplication, uniparental disomy, and imprinting related to absence of a maternal copy of a gene. The locus for the syndrome has been isolated to 11p15. A gene called IGF2 (insulin growth factor 2) has been implicated, but does not seem to explain the full range of anomalies in the syndrome.

Speech Disorders: Speech onset is often mildly delayed secondary to possible hypotonia and occasional mild developmental delay. Hypoglycemia is a common finding that can contribute to hypotonia and developmental delay. Articulation disorders are very common related to macroglossia and malocclusion. Patients with Beckwith-Wiedemann syndrome are typically prognathic and also have dental spacing abnormalities. The presence of a large tongue together with the jaw and dental anomalies results in obligatory anterior articulation errors of distortion or compensatory placement errors. The tongue may articulate in the mandibular arch rather than the maxillary arch for lingua-alveolar sounds because of the macroglossia. Cleft palate or submucous cleft palate is a fairly common finding in Beckwith-Wiedemann syndrome that can complicate the articulation disorders. Because hypotonia is also common in the syndrome, children with Beckwith-Wiedemann syndrome, who have cleft palate and velopharyngeal insufficiency, are very likely to develop compensatory patterns, including glottal stop substitutions, pharyngeal fricatives, and pharyngeal stops. Many patients with Beckwith-Wiedemann syndrome also have hypertrophic tonsils and/or adenoids, which may cause a chronic mouth-open, tongue forward posture, aggravating the macroglossia and hypotonia and resulting in fronting errors.

Feeding Disorders: Early feeding in the neonatal period is occasionally complicated by hypotonia and macroglossia. Airway obstruction is common, which may result in early failure-to-thrive.

Hearing Disorders: Chronic middle ear effusions with conductive hearing loss is common, especially in patients with cleft palate.

Voice Disorders: Hoarseness of unknown etiology has been observed in some patients.

Resonance Disorders: Hypernasality is possible in individuals with cleft palate. If hypotonia is present, hypernasality is more likely to develop. Hyponasality may also occur secondary to adenoid hypertrophy, and mixed hyper/hyponasality may also occur in patients with hypertrophic tonsils and adenoids. Oral resonance may also be impaired by hypertrophic tonsils.

Language Disorders: Language development is variable and depends on the presence or absence of cognitive impairment. Intellect is often normal, but mild impairment or borderline cognition is not uncommon.

Other Clinical Features:

Growth: overgrowth; hemihypertrophy;

Craniofacial: large mouth; mandibular prognathism; macroglossia; cleft palate;

Gastrointestinal/abdominal: omphalocele; prune belly; umbilical hernia; enlarged liver;

Metabolic/endocrine: neonatal hypoglycemia; anomalies of the renal medulla; adrenocortical cytomegaly;

Motor development: hypotonia (may be secondary to hypoglycemia);

Central nervous system: occasional cognitive impairment; seizures (not common); hydrocephalus (not common);

Genital: enlarged genitalia (male and female);

Other: development of neoplasias including Wilms' tumor; adrenal carcinoma nephroblastoma, among others; cardiomyopathy; abnormal creases on the ear lobes and indentations on the back of the ear; development of neoplasias, including Wilm's tumor.

Natural History: The neonatal period is complicated by hypotonia, which may be secondary to hypoglycemia. The hypoglycemia resolves over time and there is significant catch-up of developmental milestones. The developmental, speech, and language phenotypes improve over time, but patients must be screened frequently for the development of neoplasias, particularly Wilms' tumor. The early overgrowth eventually plateaus, and after puberty growth slows so that individuals with Beckwith-Wiedemann syndrome do not have adult gigantism.

Treatment Prognosis: The prognosis is excellent for normal speech and language.

Differential Diagnosis: Overgrowth is a feature of a number of syndromes which may also have hypotonia as an early feature, including **Sotos syndrome.** The presence of hypoglycemia and large birth size may resemble babies of diabetic mothers, a teratogenic effect. Hemihypertrophy and hemihyperplasia also exist as distinct syndromes. Omphalocele with facial anomalies and hypotonia has been reported in Shprintzen-Goldberg II syndrome.

B

Bencze Syndrome

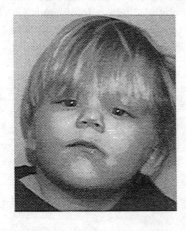

Facial asymmetry in a child with Bencze syndrome.

Also Known As: Hemifacial hyperplasia; HFH

This is a rare syndrome with the association of cleft palate (typically submucous clefts), facial asymmetry, and strabismus (esotropia). All aspects of facial growth (skeletal and soft tissue) are affected.

Major System(s) Affected: Craniofacial; ocular.

Etiology: Autosomal dominant inheritance. The gene has not yet been mapped or identified.

Speech Disorders: Malocclusion is common in the syndrome, with facial asymmetry resulting in lateral open-bite. Therefore, obligatory articulatory distortions are likely. Compensatory articulation patterns secondary to clefting may also occur.

Feeding Disorders: Feeding problems have not been reported or observed, other than the transient difficulties occasionally associated with clefting.

Hearing Disorders: Middle ear effusion secondary to cleft palate may result in intermittent conductive hearing loss. However, structural anomalies of the middle ear are not a part of the syndrome so that hearing is otherwise normal.

Voice Disorders: Voice disorders have not been reported or observed.

Resonance Disorders: Hypernasality secondary to cleft palate (or submucous cleft palate) may be found.

Language Disorders: Language disorders have not been observed or reported.

Other Clinical Features:

Craniofacial: facial asymmetry; enlargement of one side of the face, including the facial skeleton (including the zygomas and orbital rims), muscle, and glandular tissues; cleft palate (most reported cases have been submucous clefts);

Ocular: strabismus, typically esotropia; amblyopia.

Natural History: Facial asymmetry becomes more obvious with age and growth, but is not really progressive. It is simply easier to detect the asymmetry in the older and larger face. There are no late-onset anomalies.

Treatment Prognosis: Treatment of the cleft, strabismus, and facial asymmetry by surgical means has an excellent prognosis.

Differential Diagnosis: Facial asymmetry is common in a number of syndromes, including **oculo-auriculo-vertebral dysplasia** (OAV), **velo-cardio-facial syndrome** (VCFS), **Beckwith-Wiedemann syndrome, hemihypertrophy,** and **Sturge-Weber syndrome.** Bencze syndrome differs from these other syndromes because of the absence of other extracranial anomalies, or other obvious facial anomalies, such as ear tags and microtia in OAV, and port-wine birth mark in Sturge-Weber. VCFS has over 180 other anomalies, and individuals with **Beckwith-Wiedemann syndrome** have early overgrowth and hypoglycemia.

Berardinelli Syndrome

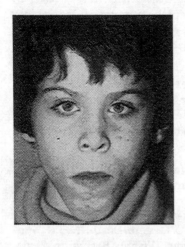

Note the triangular face and decreased buccal fat in a young child with Berardinelli syndrone.

Also Known As: Seip syndrome; lipoatrophic diabetes; congenital lipodystrophy, Berardinelli-Seip type

Berardinelli syndrome is one of a number of rare syndromes that feature severe wasting of subcutaneous fat. Cognitive impairment is common, affecting over 50% of cases.

Major System(s) Affected: Growth; craniofacial; central nervous system; liver; cardiac; renal; endocrine/metabolic; integument (skin and hair); genitourinary; musculature.

Etiology: Autosomal recessive inheritance. The gene has not yet been mapped or identified.

Speech Disorders: Articulation may be marked by fronting errors related to tonsillar hypertrophy.

Feeding Disorders: Feeding may be impaired secondary to airway obstruction caused by hypertrophic tonsils and/or adenoids. Early failure-to-thrive has been noted. Patients cannot convert food into fat and should therefore restrict meals in size so that they do not consume more calories than they need for immediate energy levels.

Hearing Disorders: Hearing loss has not been reported in association with Berardinelli syndrome.

Voice Disorders: Hoarseness is common, associated with lipodystrophy and enlarged tonsils that prompt constant postnasal drip.

Resonance Disorders: Abnormal oral resonance or mixed hyper-/hyponasality secondary to hypertrophic tonsils is common. Hyponasality related to adenoid hypertrophy may also occur.

Language Disorders: Language impairment occurs in the more than 50% of patients with cognitive impairment. The degree of cognitive impairment is variable, ranging from mild to severe.

Other Clinical Features:

Growth: progressive lipodystrophy;

Craniofacial: lack of buccal fat pads; triangular-shaped face;

Central nervous system: cognitive deficiency; hypothalamic hamartomas;

Liver: enlarged liver; cirrhosis;

Cardiac: cardiomegaly;

Renal: enlarged kidneys;

Endocrine/metabolic: elevated metabolism; diabetes mellitus; hyperglycemia;

Integument (skin and hair): thick, abundant, and curly scalp hair; acanthosis nigracans; hyperpigmentation of the skin;

Genitourinary: enlarged genitals; polycystic ovaries in females; precocious sexual maturation;

Musculature: muscle wasting.

Natural History: The subcutaneous wasting is progressive. The onset of diabetes signals a worsening of long-term prognosis, and many patients succumb to the complications of chronic diabetes in their 30s.

Treatment Prognosis: Tonsillectomy can resolve the oral resonance and articulation disorders. Language impairment and intellect are static and may therefore respond to traditional modes of therapy.

Differential Diagnosis: There are a number of syndromes with the appearance of premature senility or subcutaneous wasting, but they typically have more severe dysmorphology associated with the craniofacial structures, such as progeria and Hallerman-Streiff syndrome. Granddad syndrome has a very similar facial appearance, but does not have the endocrine and metabolic anomalies of Berardinelli syndrome. Dunnigan syndrome is similar to Berardinelli syndrome, but has multiple dental anomalies as well.

Binder Syndrome

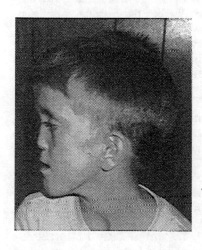

Maxillonasal dysplasia resulting in a flat facial profile, relative mandibular prognathism, and deficient midface in a 7-year-old child with Binder syndrome.

Also Known As: Maxillonasal dysplasia

Individuals with Binder syndrome have midfacial retrusion, often severe. Intellect and development are normal. Facially, they may occasionally resemble individuals with milder expressions of **Crouzon syndrome,** but craniosynostosis is not a feature of Binder syndrome.

Major System(s) Affected: Craniofacial; limb; spine.

Etiology: Unknown. Autosomal dominant inheritance and multi-factorial inheritance have been hypothesized.

Speech Disorders: Speech is marked by obligatory distortions of sounds articulated anteriorly, including lingua-alveolar and lingua-dental sounds. Tongue protrusion often occurs secondary to severe maxillary hypoplasia and anterior skeletal open-bite. Bilabial sounds may be produced with lower lip to upper dentition contact (dento-labial).

Feeding Disorders: Feeding disorders do not occur in infancy. Chewing may be somewhat im-

67

paired by malocclusion in childhood and adolescence, but feeding is not impaired.

Hearing Disorders: Hearing is typically normal.

Voice Disorders: Voice is typically normal.

Resonance Disorders: Hyponasality is common because the nasal capsule is small and nasal respiration may be compromised.

Language Disorders: Language is typically normal.

Other Clinical Features: Maxillary hypoplasia; short nose; short anterior cranial base; anterior skeletal open-bite; absence of the anterior nasal spine; minor vertebral anomalies; minor shortening of the distal phalanges of the fingers.

Natural History: Children with Binder syndrome typically appear normal at birth and during infancy. With age, the mandible grows normally, but the maxilla is deficient which is evident in early childhood, typically before 5 years of age. The maxilla shows little or no growth from childhood into adult life.

Treatment Prognosis: Orthognathic surgery can resolve the functional and aesthetic abnormalities associated with Binder syndrome. The prognosis is excellent. Treatment of the articulation impairment should be deferred until after reconstructive surgery.

Differential Diagnosis: Severe maxillary deficiency is common in many syndromes of craniosynostosis, including **Crouzon, Pfeiffer, Saethre-Chotzen,** and **Jackson-Weiss syndromes.** However, craniosynostosis does not occur in Binder syndrome. With the exception of **Crouzon syndrome,** other syndromes of craniosynostosis have distinctive patterns of limb malformation.

Blepharonasofacial Syndrome

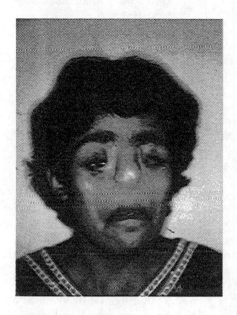

Blepharophimosis, trapezoid-shaped mouth, and tubular nose in an adolescent with blepharonasofacial syndrome.

Also Known As:

This is a rare dominantly inherited syndrome with mental retardation and craniofacial anomalies involving the eyes and mouth.

Major System(s) Affected:
Craniofacial; central nervous system.

Etiology:
Autosomal dominant inheritance. The gene has not been mapped or identified.

Speech Disorders:
Speech onset is delayed, sometimes severely. In the most severe cases, speech may not develop.

Feeding Disorders:
Feeding disorders have not been reported or observed.

Hearing Disorders:
Hearing disorders have not been reported or observed.

Voice Disorders: Voice disorders have not been reported or observed.

Resonance Disorders: Resonance may be hyponasal or have a cul-de-sac quality secondary to anterior nasal obstruction.

Language Disorders: Language is impaired in essentially all cases because of the frequent finding of cognitive impairment. Reported IQ range is 35–68.

Other Clinical Features:

    Craniofacial: large nose with a bulbous tip; telecanthus; lacrimal duct obstruction; abnormal placement of the lacrimal puncta; facial hypotonia; expressionless facial appearance;

    Central nervous system: cognitive impairment; torsion dystonia.

Natural History: The cognitive and neurologic symptoms are present throughout life and are static.

Treatment Prognosis: Surgical treatment of the eye anomalies is possible. The effects of treatment on speech and language are dependent on the severity of cognitive impairment.

Differential Diagnosis: Telecanthus or hypertelorism and cognitive impairment are found as features of blepharophimosis syndrome (mental retardation is an occasional finding), **Opitz syndrome** (an X-linked disorder), and **craniofrontonasal dysplasia syndrome.**

Bloom Syndrome

Also Known As:

Bloom syndrome is a complex autosomal recessive genetic disorder of short stature and a high frequency of cancer that involves mutable chromosomal structure. Over 20 anomalies are associated with this syndrome, which is most common among Ashkenazi Jews of Eastern European origin. Nearly 1% of Israeli Ashkenazi Jews are gene carriers. The gene is far less common in other racial and ethnic subgroups.

Major System(s) Affected:
Growth; integument; craniofacial; immune; cardiopulmonary; metabolic/endocrine; reproductive; central nervous system.

Etiology: Autosomal recessive inheritance. The gene has been mapped to 15q26.1.

Speech Disorders: Speech is typically normal, although in some cases there may be relatively late onset.

Feeding Disorders: Neonatal feeding disorders have not been documented or observed. Adult feeding disorders may develop later if neoplasias occur in the digestive tract or if general vitality is reduced by chronic illness or cancer.

Hearing Disorders: Conductive hearing loss secondary to chronic ear infections and middle ear effusions are common.

Voice Disorders: Voice is high pitched and has been described as "squeaky."

Resonance Disorders: Resonance disorders have not been reported or observed.

Language Disorders: Language development is typically normal or only slightly delayed in some cases.

Other Clinical Features:

Growth: short stature of prenatal onset; low birthweight;

Integument: telangiectasias; erythema induced by exposure to sunlight; patches of both hyperpigmentation and hypopigmentation; café-au-lait spots;

Craniofacial: micrognathia or retrognathia; malar hypoplasia; thin, triangular face; dolicocephaly; prominent nose;

Immune: chronic upper and lower respiratory infections;

Cardiopulmonary: pulmonary insufficiency; cardiomyopathy;

Metabolic/endocrine: diabetes mellitus;

Reproductive: sterility; testicular hypoplasia; cryptorchidism;

Central nervous system: learning disabilities;

Other: very high frequency of neoplasias, especially leukemia, lymphoma, and skin cancers.

Natural History: Following low birth weight, growth velocity remains steady, but height and weight remain low throughout life. Neoplasias typically develop in adolescence or early adult life. As a result of chronic infections, respiratory disorders, and the frequency of neoplasias, life expectancy is often dramatically shortened. With age, there is a high frequency of chromosome breakage and sister chromatid exchange of genetic material, which may lead to somatic mutations and the high frequency of neoplasias.

Treatment Prognosis: The administration of growth hormone has shown promise in increasing height. It is unclear if there is a positive effect on voice production, but it is likely that with increased stature and growth, vocal pitch may normalize.

Differential Diagnosis: There are a number of syndromes that show a high frequency of neoplasias in association with short stature, immune disorders, and skin lesions, including **Cockayne syndrome** and Rothmund-Thompson syndrome. Unlike Bloom syndrome, **Cockayne syndrome** is marked by severe cognitive impairment with rapid deterioration in adult life. Rothmund-Thompson syndrome has significant limb anomalies (such as severely hypoplastic thumbs) and dental anomalies.

BOF Syndrome

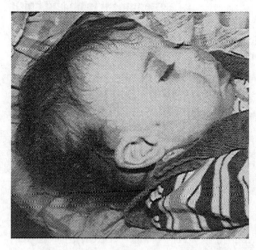

BOF syndrome:
Note shortening of the
midline of the upper lip.

Also Known As: Branchioocu-lofacial syndrome; BOFS

This is a rare syndrome with distinctive facial findings including a shortened and notched upper lip that appears to be cleft, but is not. There are also prominent branchial clefts in the postauricular area bilaterally, which may be accented by hemangiomas. The lip is marked by a short philtrum and may also have a prominent midline labial frenulum.

Major System(s) Affected: Craniofacial; ocular; growth; dental; integument (skin and hair).

Etiology: Autosomal dominant inheritance. The gene has not been mapped or identified.

Speech Disorders: Anterior distortions of bilabial sounds and obligatory placement errors may be caused by the shortening of the upper lip. Dental anomalies may also add to the articulatory distortions.

Feeding Disorders: Neonatal feeding disorders secondary to cleft palate may occur.

Hearing Disorders: Mild conductive hearing loss is a possible finding.

Voice Disorders: Voice disorders have not been reported or observed.

Resonance Disorders: Hypernasality secondary to cleft palate may occur.

Language Disorders: Language development is typically normal. Cognition is normal.

Other Clinical Features:

Craniofacial: pseudocleft of the upper lip; protuberant lower lip; lip pits; branchial clefts; hemangiomas of the branchial clefts; broad nasal bridge; flat nasal tip;

Ocular: strabismus; ocular coloboma (iris, retina, optic nerve); orbital hemangiomas; nasolacrimal duct obstruction;

Growth: low birthweight; relative short stature;

Dental: tooth anomalies;

Integument (skin and hair): hemangiomas; scalp cysts; premature graying of the scalp hair.

Natural History: Postnatal growth tends to be slow. Intellect has been normal in the majority of patients. There are no major late-onset anomalies.

Treatment Prognosis: Surgical correction of the physical anomalies is possible. Speech correction is also possible following surgical correction, or compensatory placements can be taught to accommodate for oral anomalies.

Differential Diagnosis: Branchial clefts or sinuses are found in a number of other syndromes, the most common of which is **BOR syndrome** (branchio-oto-renal syndrome, or Melnick-Fraser syndrome). However, BOR syndrome has significant mixed or sensorineural hearing loss as a common finding and does not feature a midline lip abnormality. Lip pits are a common feature of **van der Woude syndrome** and **popliteal pterygium syndrome**.

BOR Syndrome

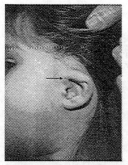

Figure 1: Arrow shows preauricular pit in BOR syndrome.

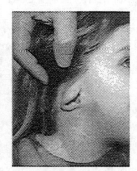

Figure 2: Overfolded auricle for the opposite ear.

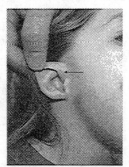

Figure 3: Arrow shows preauricular pit after the ear is reflected back.

Also Known As: Branchio-oto-renal syndrome; Melnick-Fraser syndrome

BOR syndrome is a relatively common multiple anomaly disorder that shows phenotypic overlap with a number of other common disorders and has been misdiagnosed in many cases. Recognition of the syndrome is important because of the renal malformations that accompany the hearing loss and structural anomalies of the ear.

Major System(s) Affected: Auditory; craniofacial; renal; neck; pulmonary.

Etiology: Autosomal dominant inheritance. The gene has been mapped to the long arm of chromosome 8, at 8q13.3.

Speech Disorders: Speech may be affected by mixed or sensorineural hearing loss. Cleft palate (often submucous) is also found in some cases and may lead to compensatory articulation disorders. Malocclusion, including anterior skeletal open-bite, lateral open-bite, or retrognathia is a fairly common finding, which may result in obligatory distortions or substitutions.

Feeding Disorders: Feeding disorders in infancy have not been considered a feature of BOR syndrome. There are no feeding impairments in childhood, adolescence, or adult life.

Hearing Disorders: Hearing loss is probably the most common manifestation of BOR syndrome and may be purely conductive, mixed, or sensorineural. Ear malformations are common in BOR, including anomalies of the external ear, external ear canal, middle ear, cochlea, and vestibular system. The most frequent type of hearing loss in BOR is mixed because both conductive and sensorineural deficits are common. The degree of impairment ranges from mild to profound and is usually symmetric, but asymmetric cases have been seen. Hypoplasia of the apex of the cochlea has been documented in many cases, as has fixation of the footplate of the stapes.

Voice Disorders: Voice is typically normal in BOR.

Resonance Disorders: Resonance may be abnormal based on the effects of sensorineural hearing loss and/or cleft palate. Cleft palate in BOR is most often submucous,

and is, therefore, not detected in many cases.

Language Disorders: Language is typically normal in BOR, other than the effects of the more severe forms of hearing loss in some cases.

Other Clinical Features:

Auditory: external ear malformations, typically small cup-shaped ears, or lop ears; ossicular anomalies, including stapes fixation; hypoplastic cochlear apex; vestibular anomalies; ear pits;

Craniofacial: micrognathia; retrognathia; facial asymmetry; dental malocclusion; cleft palate;

Renal: small or absent kidneys; cystic kidneys; anomalies of the renal collecting system;

Neck: branchial clefts;

Pulmonary: pulmonary hypoplasia.

Natural History: The hearing loss in BOR syndrome is typically static, but several cases of mildly progressive hearing loss have been observed. Cognition and motor development are normal. Early detection of kidney anomalies is important and treatment of the kidney problems associated with the malformations is possible.

Treatment Prognosis: Speech therapy, amplification, and surgical management are all expected to have positive outcomes in the large majority of cases.

Differential Diagnosis: The presence of external ear anomalies associated with ear pits, hearing loss, and facial asymmetry is a common combination in BOR and is often mistaken for **oculo-auriculo-vertebral dysplasia** (OAV, or hemifacial microsomia). Because of this common diagnostic mistake, for many years children born with OAV (hemifacial microsomia) were often referred for examination of the kidneys and the collecting system (often with intravenous pyelograms). In true cases of OAV, positive findings would be rare, but in patients with BOR, renal anomalies are common. There are a number of rare syndromes of hearing loss with the association of ear pits and sensorineural hearing loss with other minor malformations, but the most common syndrome to be suspected should be BOR.

Börjeson-Forssman-Lehmann Syndrome

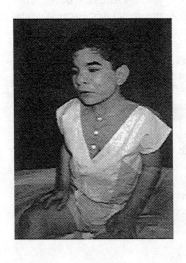

Note the coarse facial features, large ears, and microcephaly associated with Börjeson-Forssman-Lehmann syndrome.

Also Known As: Börjeson syndrome

Börjeson-Forssman-Lehmann syndrome is a rare X-linked recessive disorder characterized by mental retardation, usually severe, a characteristic facial appearance, and abnormal metabolism and secondary sexual characteristics.

Major System(s) Affected: Central nervous system; craniofacial; endocrine/metabolic; limbs.

Etiology: X-linked recessive inheritance. The gene has been mapped to Xq26-27.

Speech Disorders: Most patients with Börjeson-Forssman-Lehmann syndrome do not develop significant amounts of language or speech. Those who do, have dysarthric speech with marked reduction of length of utterance.

Feeding Disorders: Feeding disorders have not been reported or observed.

78

Hearing Disorders: Hearing is typically normal.

Voice Disorders: Voice is high pitched and hoarse.

Resonance Disorders: Resonance disorders have not been reported or observed.

Language Disorders: Language is severely impaired or does not develop.

Other Clinical Features:

Central nervous system: mental retardation, usually severe; seizures;

Craniofacial: coarse facies; prominent supraorbital ridges; puffy upper eyelids; ptosis; puffy facial soft tissues; large ears;

Endocrine/metabolic: slow basal metabolism; obesity; short stature; small male genitals; gynecomastia;

Limbs: small digits; tapered fingers; wide-spaced toes.

Natural History: The developmental impairment and growth deficiency is evident in infancy. The obesity and gynecomastia become more pronounced following the onset of puberty.

Treatment Prognosis: Poor.

Differential Diagnosis: Obesity and cognitive impairment are common in **Prader-Willi syndrome,** the **Bardet-Biedl syndromes,** and **Laurence-Moon syndrome.** However, the facial appearance is distinctive in Börjeson-Forssman-Lehmann syndrome, which will distinguish the disorder from other syndromes of obesity with cognitive impairment. The facial appearance is similar to that found in **Coffin-Lowry syndrome,** but the latter syndrome does not have the endocrine and metabolic findings associated with Börjeson-Forssman-Lehmann syndrome.

Brachial Plexus Neuropathy

Also Known As: Neuritis with brachial predilection; recurrent brachial plexus neuropathy with cleft palate

This syndrome is marked initially by cleft palate, but is distinctive because of its late-onset findings. Sudden attacks of shoulder pain usually begin in childhood with a progression of neurologic symptoms, including parasthesia and muscle weakness.

Major System(s) Affected: Neurologic; craniofacial; limbs; skeletal.

Etiology: Autosomal dominant inheritance. The gene has been mapped to 17q24-q25.

Speech Disorders: Individuals with clefts may have compensatory articulation patterns. If, however, there is no evidence of velopharyngeal insufficiency, speech is usually normal.

Feeding Disorders: Feeding may be complicated by cleft palate, but is otherwise normal.

Hearing Disorders: Conductive hearing loss secondary to middle ear effusion is common in early childhood secondary to cleft palate, but hearing is otherwise normal.

Voice Disorders: Hoarseness.

Resonance Disorders: Hypernasality may be present secondary to cleft palate.

Language Disorders: Language is normal.

Other Clinical Features:

Neurologic: brachial neuritis; parasthesia over the arms and hands; muscle weakness; reduced reflexes;

Craniofacial: cleft palate (often submucous cleft); facial asymmetry; deep-set eyes; hypotelorism; vertical maxillary excess; small mouth; facial paresis;

Limbs: muscle wasting; syndactyly;

Skeletal: winged scapulae.

Natural History: Other than cleft palate, the presentation at birth is typically normal. The onset of neurologic symptoms typically begins near school age, starting with sharp unexplained pain in the shoulder area. The disorder progresses to a loss of sensation in the arms (parasthesia) followed by muscle weakness and then muscle atrophy. At about the same time, the voice begins to become hoarse.

Treatment Prognosis: The speech disorders must be treated symptomatically. The voice disorder may be related to recurrent laryngeal nerve dysfunction.

Differential Diagnosis: Progressive neuropathy is seen in a number of autosomal recessive disorders, such as Refsum syndrome, but are typically associated with skin lesions and a more severe global neurologic picture.

C Syndrome

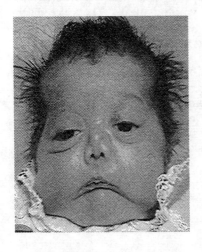

C syndrome: Note severe craniofacial anomalies, including trigonocephaly and proptosis.

Also Known As: Opitz trigonocephaly syndrome

This is a rare autosomal recessive disorder with distinctive craniofacial anomalies, limb disorders, and mental retardation in those individuals who survive the neonatal period. Half or more of affected infants do not survive to childhood.

Major System(s) Affected: Craniofacial; limb; central nervous system; skeletal; cardiac; skin; genitals; ocular.

Etiology: Autosomal recessive inheritance. The gene has not been mapped or identified.

Speech Disorders: The cognitive impairment in C syndrome is severe and the development of speech is unlikely.

Feeding Disorders: Early failure-to-thrive is common and may be related to a number of factors including severe hypotonia, airway obstruction, and heart anomalies.

Hearing Disorders: Hearing impairment has not been reported, but conductive hearing loss is likely related to craniofacial anomalies.

Voice Disorders: Voice has not been assessed because of the lack of speech and language development.

Resonance Disorders: Resonance has not been assessed because of the lack of speech and language development.

Language Disorders: The cognitive impairment in C syndrome is severe and the development of expressive or receptive language is unlikely.

Other Clinical Features:

Craniofacial: trigonocephaly; metopic synostosis; microcephaly; upslanting eyes; depressed nasal root; epicanthal folds; micrognathia; posteriorly rotated ears; multiple oral frenula; soft tissue hypertrophy of the palatal shelves; broad maxillary alveolus; abnormal helical rims; occasional cleft palate;

Limb: polydactyly; syndactyly; short limbs; joint contractures; talipes equinovarus; joint dislocations;

Central nervous system: severe mental retardation; hypotonia; seizures;

Skeletal: short neck; hip dysplasia;

Cardiac: heart malformations;

Skin: lax skin;

Genitals: cryptorchidism; prominent clitoris in females;

Ocular: strabismus.

Natural History: Head circumference and shape are normal at birth. Microcephaly and craniofacial growth anomalies progress after birth. Limb and joint abnormalities are evident from birth, and performance is impaired from birth. Approximately 50% of known cases have not survived infancy.

Treatment Prognosis: Poor.

Differential Diagnosis: A number of chromosomal rearrangement syndromes have trigonocephaly and microcephaly as common findings, including del(9p), del(llq), and dup(13q).

Campomelic Dysplasia

Also Known As: Campomelic syndrome; campomelic dwarfism

Campomelic dysplasia is a rare syndrome of short stature with a low frequency of survival past infancy. It is important to recognize because of the implications for feeding difficulties in affected neonates. The few infants who have survived have been severely retarded. Birth frequency is approximately 1:100,000. Although originally suspected to be inherited as an autosomal recessive disorder, there was a strong prevalence of females to males, approximately 3:1. It was found that many of the phenotypically female infants were cytogenetically male (46XY). It is now known that the syndrome is an autosomal dominant disorder caused by a deletion from the long arm of chromosome 17.

Major System(s) Affected: Growth; craniofacial; skeletal; limbs; pulmonary; central nervous system; genitals.

Etiology: Autosomal dominant expression based on haploinsufficiency of 17q24.3-q25.1. The syndrome is probably a contiguous gene syndrome. Sex reversal is related to a gene, SOX9, which is adjacent to the chromosomal breakpoint.

Speech Disorders: The large majority of patients diagnosed with campomelic dysplasia do not survive infancy because of severe respiratory complications, including Robin sequence, tracheal ring anomalies, and pulmonary hypoplasia. Therefore, opportunities to observe speech have been limited. However, a high percentage of surviving individuals have severe mental retardation and do not develop speech. It may be presumed that patients who do develop speech have articulation impairment based on malocclusion and the secondary effects of cleft palate.

Feeding Disorders: Early failure-to-thrive is the rule based on severe multifactorial airway compromise. Airway obstruction may be caused by micrognathia, pulmonary hypoplasia, tracheal ring anomalies, and hypotonia. None of these findings are mutually exclusive and many patients have all of these anomalies simultaneously. In cases with this severity of abnormality, feeding cannot be successful if the airway problems are insurmountable.

Hearing Disorders: Hearing loss has not been specifically identified, but conductive impairment secondary to clefting and chronic middle ear effusion can be presumed.

Voice Disorders: The cry of affected infants is typically weak, probably secondary to pulmonary insufficiency.

Resonance Disorders: Clefting is typically of the Robin type (very wide). Therefore, velopharyngeal insufficiency is possible, if not likely, in surviving infants.

Language Disorders: Language impairment is typically severe in surviving individuals.

Other Clinical Features:

Growth: small stature;

Craniofacial: Robin sequence; severe micrognathia; hypertelorism; depressed nasal root; cleft palate;

Skeletal: abnormal pelvis; hip dislocation; kyphoscoliosis; hypoplastic scapulae; 11 rib pairs;

Limbs: curved upper limbs; short phalanges in both the hands and feet; bowing of the femur; talipes equinovarus;

Pulmonary: pulmonary hypoplasia;

Central nervous system: mental retardation, hypotonia; absent olfactory tracts;

Genitals: male sex reversal.

Natural History: The majority of affected individuals die in the neonatal period or infancy. Those who survive tend to be severely impaired. Some cases with milder expression have been reported.

Treatment Prognosis: Typically poor.

Differential Diagnosis: Curved limbs are found in several skeletal dysplasias.

Cardiofaciocutaneous Syndrome

Also Known As: CFC syndrome

Cardiofaciocutaneous syndrome is a rare syndrome of mental retardation that includes heart anomalies and skin disorders, classified by some clinicians as a cardiocutaneous syndrome. The syndrome may be underdetected because its features overlap with several other rare syndromes with similar manifestations. The syndrome, or at least some cases clinically diagnosed with CFC, may be allelic with **Noonan syndrome.** This means that a different form of the gene that causes **Noonan syndrome** may also cause at least some cases of CFC.

Major System(s) Affected: Central nervous system; cardiac; growth; integument (skin/hair); craniofacial; ocular.

Etiology: Autosomal dominant inheritance. Some cases have been linked to a gene mapped to 12q24.

Speech Disorders: Articulation is often impaired secondary to poor oral coordination. Mild dysarthria is seen occasionally.

Feeding Disorders: Early hypotonia may impair early attempts at nursing.

Hearing Disorders: Hearing is typically normal.

Voice Disorders: Voice disorders have not been reported or observed.

Resonance Disorders: Resonance disorders have not been reported or observed.

Language Disorders: Language is uniformly delayed and impaired secondary to global cognitive impairment.

Other Clinical Features:

    Central nervous system: mental retardation;

    Cardiac: atrial septal defect; pulmonic stenosis; cardiomyopathy;

Growth: short stature;

Integument (skin/hair): sparse brittle hair; hyperkeratosis; ichthyosis; thin fingernails;

Craniofacial: macrocephaly; bitemporal depressions; high forehead; depressed nasal root; posteriorly rotated ears, protuberant auricles;

Ocular: nystagmus, downslanting palpebral fissures;

Other: pectus excavatum or carinatum; prominent fingertip pads.

Natural History: The cognitive impairments in CFC are static and present from birth. The skin anomalies are progressive. Short stature is of postnatal onset.

Treatment Prognosis: Limitations in performance persist and may limit the progress in speech and language treatment.

Differential Diagnosis: The craniofacial manifestations resemble those in **Noonan syndrome.** Macrocephaly with skin lesions are common in **neurofibromatosis, type I** (von Recklinghausen type).

Carpenter Syndrome

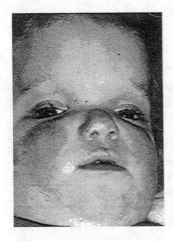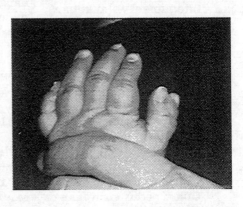

Craniosynostosis, depressed nasal root, maxillary hypoplasia (left) and preaxial polydactyly (right) in Carpenter syndrome.

Also Known As: Acrocephalopolysyndactyly; acrocephalopolysyndactyly type II

Major System(s) Affected: Craniofacial; limbs; central nervous system; cardiac; growth; genitals.

Carpenter syndrome is a well known but rare syndrome of craniosynostosis. Fewer than 50 cases have been reported in the medical literature, but it is likely that many more cases have been seen and misdiagnosed. Although the association of craniosynostosis and limb anomalies is common, the hand and foot abnormalities in Carpenter syndrome are distinctive and not similar to those found in **Apert, Pfeiffer, Jackson-Weiss,** or **Saethre-Chotzen syndromes.**

Etiology: Autosomal recessive inheritance. The gene has not been mapped or identified yet.

Speech Disorders: Speech production is variable, ranging from normal to severely impaired based on cognitive status and the degree of craniofacial malformation. Articulation is often impaired by malocclusion which may include anterior skeletal open-bite, Class III malocclusion, and in some cases a Class II malocclusion with deep overbite.

Feeding Disorders: Early feeding may be impaired by hypotonia in patients with significant neurologic involvement.

Hearing Disorders: Hearing is typically normal. But on occasion there may be a mild conductive hearing loss relative to middle ear effusion because of poor eustachian tube function.

Voice Disorders: Voice disorders have not been reported or observed.

Resonance Disorders: Both hyponasality and mild hypernasality have been observed in some cases. The author has seen one patient with hypernasality and a submucous cleft palate.

Language Disorders: Language is delayed and impaired in essentially all cases with cognitive impairment (the majority of known cases).

Other Clinical Features:

Craniofacial: craniosynostosis involving multiple sutures; downslanting palpebral fissures; occasional kleeblattschadel; asymmetric cranium; constricted maxillary arch; occasional micrognathia; telecanthus or hypertelorism;

Limbs: preaxial polydactyly more commonly of the feet, but also of the hands; syndactyly;

Central nervous system: mental retardation in most cases, but normal intellect has been observed;

Cardiac: conotruncal heart anomalies have been found in approximately 30% of cases, including tetralogy of Fallot, VSD, ASD, and pulmonic stenosis;

Growth: the majority of cases have been of relatively short stature;

Genitals: hypogonadism;

Other: short neck.

Natural History: Birth weight is typically normal. Head shape may be relatively normal at birth, but evidence of craniosynostosis becomes evident shortly after birth and head shape may be severely abnormal. In many cases, there is asymmetric synostosis resulting in marked cranial asymmetry. Cognitive deficiency is not typically related to the synostosis, although failure to surgically treat cranial fusions may result in increased intracranial pressure. However, cognitive deficiency often occurs even after craniosynostosis has been surgically resolved.

Treatment Prognosis: Surgical treatment of the skull anomalies is indicated and can be very successful. The cognitive deficiency is static and should respond to appropriate treatment up to the limitations of the presumed CNS anomalies.

Differential Diagnosis: The cranial anomalies in Carpenter syndrome do not really resemble those typically seen in **Crouzon, Apert, Pfeiffer, Jackson-Weiss,** or **Saethre-Chotzen syndromes,** but the association of limb and cranial anomalies may lead some clinicians to suspect these syndromes. Polydactyly is a common manifestation of the oral-facial-digital syndromes, which may also have marked craniofacial anomalies, although craniosynostosis is not a common finding in the **OFD syndromes.**

Cartilage-Hair Hypoplasia

Also Known As: Metaphyseal chondrodysplasia, McKusick type; CHH

CHH is a syndrome of short stature and ectodermal dysplasia (anomalies of the hair, skin, and dentition) that was originally identified in an Amish population and then subsequently also identified in the Finnish. It is not unusual for an autosomal recessive genetic disorder to be largely isolated to specific ethnic, racial, or geographical subgroups.

Major System(s) Affected: Growth; integument (skin/hair/nails); dentition; gut; skeletal; limbs; craniofacial; blood; immune.

Etiology: Autosomal recessive inheritance with incomplete penetrance. The gene has been mapped to 9p13.

Speech Disorders: Articulation distortions are obligatory and related to dental abnormalities.

Feeding Disorders: Feeding disorders are not a feature of the syndrome.

Hearing Disorders: Hearing is typically normal.

Voice Disorders: Voice is occasionally hoarse.

Resonance Disorders: Resonance is normal.

Language Disorders: Language development and intellect are normal.

Other Clinical Features:

Growth: prenatal growth deficiency resulting in short stature at birth through adult life;

Integument (skin/hair/nails): skin hypopigmentation; sparse hair; fragile hair; light colored hair;

Dentition: small teeth; notched incisors;

Gut: malabsorption; celiac syndrome; Hirschsprung aganglionic megacolon; anal stenosis; esophageal atresia;

Skeletal: chondrodysplasia; lumbar lordosis; flared lower rib cage; prominent sternum; short tibias with mild bowing; short vertebrae;

Limbs: short digits (brachydactyly); small hands; limitation of bend at elbows; hyperextensible fingers;

Craniofacial: brachycephaly;

Blood: anemia; leukopenia; neutropenia; lymphopenia;

Immune: immunodeficiency; particular susceptibility to varicella and viral hepatitis; T-cell deficiency;

Other: tendency toward certain malignancies, including Hodgkin's lymphoma and leukemia.

Natural History: Birth length and weight are typically below normal limits, but become proportionately smaller with age. Although the short stature is mainly due to short limbs, the torso may also be slightly short secondary to spinal anomalies. Sparse hair extends to body hair, facial hair, and eyebrows. Microscopic examination of the hair shows it to be reduced in diameter. The blood and immune disorders become obvious with age.

Treatment Prognosis: The prognosis is typically good.

Differential Diagnosis: There are a number of other chondrodysplasias, including the Schmid type and Conradi-Hünerman syndrome. The hair anomalies and immune disorders clearly distinguish CHH from these other syndromes.

Cat Eye Syndrome

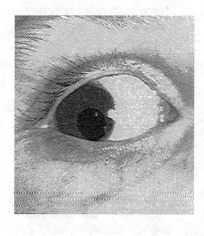

Iris coloboma in a patient with cat eye syndrome.

Also Known As: CES; chromosome 22 partial tetrasomy; inv dup(22)(q11); Schmid-Fraccaro syndrome

Cat eye syndrome is a disorder caused by a chromosomal rearrangement in the same region that causes velo-cardio-facial syndrome, 22q11. Although the chromosome region is the same as in VCFS, the syndrome is distinctly different. The term "cat eye" was originally applied as a description of the iris coloboma that is a common feature in this syndrome.

Major System(s) Affected: Central nervous system; ocular; craniofacial; ears; cardiac; gastrointestinal; renal.

Etiology: Individuals with cat eye syndrome have extra chromosome material, which is seen as a "marker" chromosome on karyotyping. The marker chromosome consists of the acrocentric short arm and a portion of the long arm of chromosome 22 to the q11 band. These markers have been demonstrated to be dicentric (two centromeres).

Speech Disorders: Speech is affected by delayed motor development and incoordination which is variable from mild to severe. Cleft palate is also a common finding (at least 25% of cases) and can result in velopharyngeal insufficiency with compensatory articulation patterns.

Feeding Disorders: Early feeding may be impaired by hypotonia. Long term, there is no major feeding problem.

Hearing Disorders: Mild conductive hearing loss is seen occasionally related to minor ear anomalies with resulting narrowing of the external canal or chronic middle ear effusions secondary to cleft palate.

Voice Disorders: Voice disorders have not been reported.

Resonance Disorders: Hypernasality is common in cases with cleft palate.

Language Disorders: Language is typically delayed, usually mildly, although in cases with more severe cognitive impairment, a moderate to severe disorder is possible.

Other Clinical Features:

Central nervous system: cognitive impairment is common, ranging from borderline to moderate, although some cases with normal intellect have been documented;

Ocular: iris coloboma in at least 70%; microphthalmia;

Ears: small ears; protuberant ears; preauricular tags or pits;

Cardiac: tetralogy of Fallot; total anomalous pulmonary venous return;

Gastrointestinal: anal atresia or abnormal anal placement; malrotation of the gut; Meckel diverticulum;

Renal: hypoplastic or aplastic kidneys, unilateral or bilateral.

Natural History: The anomalies associated with cat eye syndrome are essentially static and late-onset findings have not been noted. Growth is typically normal, although some cases have mild postnatal growth deficiency.

Treatment Prognosis: The prognosis is dependent on the degree of cognitive impairment. Some infants with cat eye syndrome do not survive the neonatal period because of heart or renal anomalies, but the majority of patients do survive and have a normal life span.

Differential Diagnosis: Ocular coloboma associated with ear anomalies, anal anomalies, and cognitive impairment is common in **CHARGE association** and may also be seen in **velo-cardio-facial syndrome.**

C

Catel-Manzke Syndrome

Also Known As: Palatodigital syndrome

Catel-Manzke syndrome is a rare syndrome with the association of Robin sequence and digital anomalies. The etiology has been reported to be X-linked recessive, but several female cases have been reported, which cast doubt on an X-linked mode of inheritance.

Major System(s) Affected: Craniofacial; limbs; cardiac.

Etiology: Unknown. X-linked recessive inheritance has been hypothesized, but female cases have been reported, and the author has seen one female newborn, suggesting that the disorder is autosomal.

Speech Disorders: Micrognathia is a common feature leading to a Class II malocclusion and obligatory placement errors. Cleft palate may also lead to compensatory articulation patterns.

Feeding Disorders: Early failure-to-thrive is an outcome of upper airway obstruction and Robin sequence. Cleft palate complicates feeding in relation to Robin sequence, but the feeding problem is primarily related to airway obstruction.

Hearing Disorders: Conductive hearing loss secondary to middle ear effusion is to be expected.

Voice Disorders: Voice disorders have not been reported or observed.

Resonance Disorders: Hypernasality secondary to cleft palate is possible.

Language Disorders: Language development is typically normal.

Other Clinical Features:

> **Craniofacial:** Robin sequence; micrognathia; cleft palate;

> **Limbs:** extra bone at the base of the index finger; ulnar deviation of the index finger; club foot;

Cardiac: ventriculoseptal defect.

Natural History: The presence of Robin sequence at birth can lead to serious airway obstruction and failure-to-thrive in early life, but with treatment and/or growth, the problem will resolve. There are no late-onset disorders associated with the syndrome.

Treatment Prognosis: There are a number of effective treatments for Robin sequence and upper airway obstruction. With palatal repair and hand surgery, the anomalies associated with Catel-Manzke syndrome can be resolved.

Differential Diagnosis: Limb anomalies associated with Robin sequence occur in a number of syndromes, including **velo-cardio-facial syndrome** (slender, tapered digits), **Freeman-Sheldon syndrome** (ulnar deviation of all digits), **distal arthrogryposis** (contractures), **otopalatodigital syndrome** (prominent finger pads), **Nager syndrome** (missing or hypoplastic thumbs), **fetal alcohol syndrome** (short digits), fetal hydantoin syndrome (absent nails and short fingers), and **de Lange syndrome** (hypoplastic digits). None of these syndromes has the accessory bone found in Catel-Manzke syndrome.

Cerebrocostomandibular Syndrome

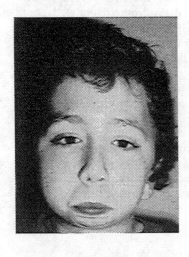

Cerebrocostomandibular syndrome: Note severe micrognathia.

Also Known As: Rib gap defects with micrognathia; rib gap syndrome

Cerebrocostomandibular syndrome is a multiple anomaly disorder associated with Robin sequence with distinctive rib anomalies. In many of the earliest documented cases, neonatal death occurred secondary to respiratory failure, but a sufficient number of cases have survived the neonatal period to establish eventual cognitive outcomes. In some cases, the palate is so severely deficient of tissue that the velum appears to be absent or nearly absent.

Major System(s) Affected: Craniofacial; skeletal; growth; central nervous system.

Etiology: Unknown. Both autosomal dominant and autosomal recessive inheritance have been hypothesized.

Speech Disorders: There are severe articulation disorders related to the micrognathia. There is little room for the tongue, which is typically small, to articulate in the oral cavity because of the severe Class II malocclusion. Tongue backing is common. Compensatory articulation secondary to cleft palate is also to be expected.

Feeding Disorders: Severe respiratory compromise leads to failure-to-thrive in the large majority of cases. Although the palatal cleft may be wide and further complicate the feeding process, the primary cause of difficulty is airway obstruction from micrognathia and glossoptosis.

Hearing Disorders: Conductive hearing impairment secondary to middle ear effusion may be anticipated in cases with cleft palate.

Voice Disorders: Voice disorders have not been reported or observed.

Resonance Disorders: Resonance is often very abnormal with a combined hypernasality and unusual muffled oral resonance pattern caused by severe micrognathia.

Language Disorders: Language may be severely impaired in cases with cognitive deficiency. Even in cases with normal intellect, the expressive language skills may lag somewhat behind receptive levels because of the airway disorders in infancy.

Other Clinical Features:

Craniofacial: severe micrognathia; cleft palate, usually severe;

Skeletal: gaps between the ribs and their vertebral junctions (costovertebral junction); other rib anomalies;

Growth: postnatal growth deficiency;

Central nervous system: mental retardation has been reported in a substantial percentage of cases, but it is unclear if this is a primary anomaly or secondary to early hypoxic brain damage.

Natural History: Respiratory distress is noted immediately after birth and persists unless treatment is applied. With age and growth, respiratory failure sometimes resolves spontaneously, but most cases require intervention.

Treatment Prognosis: Palate repair is extremely difficult in some cases because of the severe deficiency of tissue and the concern for airway compromise. Articulation errors are largely obligatory because of the severe malformation of the mandible. Speech therapy is therefore very difficult because of the orofacial structural anomalies.

Differential Diagnosis: Severe mandibular and palatal anomalies are also found in **Nager syndrome** and **Treacher Collins syndrome,** but neither of these conditions has the same rib anomalies, and the facial anomalies are different.

Cerebrooculofacioskeletal Syndrome

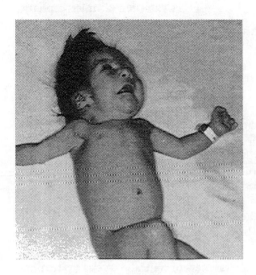

Cerebrooculofacio-skeletal syndrome (COFS): Infant with microcephaly, micrognathia, contractures, and upslanting eyes.

Also Known As: COFS; Pena-Shokeir syndrome, type II

This multiple anomaly disorder was initially named Pena-Shokeir syndrome, type II, because of some phenotypic overlap with Pena-Shokeir syndrome, but using the similar designation for two separate and distinct disorders can be confusing and lead one to believe that there is some causal link between the disorders. This rare syndrome results in severe retardation and shortened life span.

Major System(s) Affected: Central nervous system; growth; craniofacial; ocular; musculoskeletal.

Etiology: Autosomal recessive inheritance. The gene has not been mapped or identified, but there is suspicion that it may be located at either 1q23 or 16q13 because of a

101

documented case of a balanced translocation and the possibility that a gene was interrupted at one of the break points.

Speech Disorders: Speech does not develop.

Feeding Disorders: Failure-to-thrive is a constant feature.

Hearing Disorders: Hearing loss has not been documented.

Voice Disorders: Voice disorders have not been documented.

Resonance Disorders: Resonance disorders have not been documented.

Language Disorders: There is essentially no receptive or expressive language development.

Other Clinical Features:

    Central nervous system: severe cognitive impairment; hypotonia; absent corpus callosum; cerebellar hypoplasia;

Growth: low birth weight; severe growth deficiency; failure to thrive;

Craniofacial: microcephaly; large ears; prominent nasal root; micrognathia;

Ocular: microphthalmia; up-slanting eyes; cataracts;

Musculoskeletal: kyphoscoliosis; joint contractures; arthrogryposis; rocker-bottom feet; hip dislocation; osteoporosis; short neck; wide-spaced nipples.

Natural History: Following low birth weight and small size, growth becomes more deficient over time. Failure to thrive is caused by both severe central nervous system impairment and micrognathia with airway obstruction. There is progressive CNS deterioration and death usually occurs before 5 years of age.

Treatment Prognosis: Extremely poor.

Differential Diagnosis: Pena-Shokeir syndrome.

CHARGE Association

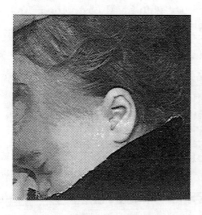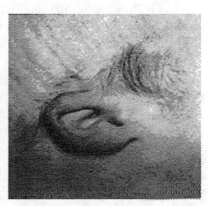

Variation in ear anomalies associated with CHARGE.

Also Known As:

CHARGE is an acronym for *Co*loboma, *H*eart anomalies, *A*tresia choanae, *R*etarded growth and development, *G*enital hypoplasia, and *E*ar anomalies. The term "association" refers an etiologically nonspecific disorder that does not show clear evidence of being a sequence. Although a number of other syndromes have anomalies that fit the CHARGE acronym, there does seem to be a core of individuals with a consistent pattern that probably does represent a distinct recurrent pattern syndrome.

Major System(s) Affected:

Central nervous system; craniofacial; growth; ocular; auditory; cardiac; skeletal; genital.

Etiology:

The large majority of cases have been sporadic occurrences, but autosomal dominant inheritance has been observed. A number of syndromes with known causation have clinical features consistent with CHARGE association, including **velo-cardio-facial syndrome** and **Wolf-Hirschhorn syndrome**.

Speech Disorders:

Speech is almost always abnormal with multifactorial contribution to poor speech production. Articulation is impaired both by malocclusion and central nervous system impairment. Sensorineural hearing loss also adds to the mix of factors that results in unintelligible speech.

Feeding Disorders: Feeding is almost always impaired by multiple factors, including choanal atresia, hypotonia, developmental delay, and congenital heart anomalies. Some children have severe failure to thrive unless the cause(s) of the feeding difficulty is identified and resolved.

Hearing Disorders: Conductive, sensorineural, and mixed hearing loss have all been observed. In many cases, a trough-shaped mixed hearing loss is common, often affecting the speech frequencies most severely. Vestibular anomalies are also common.

Voice Disorders: Hoarse or breathy voice is common and may be related to unilateral vocal fold paresis.

Resonance Disorders: Hyponasality is common, related to choanal atresia. In cases with cleft palate, there may be a mixed hyper-/hyponasality, or a cul-de-sac resonance pattern related to the combination of velopharyngeal insufficiency with nasal obstruction. An abnormal oral resonance is also common related to a short neck, small mouth, and hearing loss.

Language Disorders: Language impairment is very common and is often severe. Verbal language may not be obtained by a significant percentage of patients because of the combination of cognitive impairment and hearing loss.

Other Clinical Features:

Central nervous system: cognitive impairment; brain malformations;

Craniofacial: facial paresis; facial asymmetry; microcephaly; low-set posteriorly rotated ears; protuberant ears; prominent nasal root; microsotomia; cleft palate; occasional cleft lip; micrognathia;

Growth: short stature;

Ocular: iris, choroid, retina, and/or optic nerve coloboma; microphthalmia;

Auditory: Mondini anomaly; semicircular canal hypoplasia;

Cardiac: heart anomalies, often conotruncal, but also endocardial cushion defect;

Skeletal: short neck; scoliosis;

Genital: small phallus in males; cryptorchidism; hypospadias;

Other: occasional anal anomalies, occasional renal anomalies; tracheoesophageal fistula has been reported in a few cases.

Natural History: Birth weight is often slightly low, and postnatal growth is slow resulting in progressive short stature. All developmental milestones are delayed and language and speech are particularly impaired. The cognitive delays are static, but may be severe in some cases.

Treatment Prognosis: Variable, depending on the severity of the cognitive impairment. Surgically resolving the choanal atresia often fails because it is difficult to maintain nasal patency. Children with CHARGE tend to be chronic mouth breathers.

Differential Diagnosis: Because the CHARGE symptoms are common in other syndromes and CHARGE is considered to be etiologically heterogenous, the diagnosis of CHARGE should not rule out a syndromic diagnosis, as well. For example, children with **velocardio-facial syndrome** have been reported to have many or all of the CHARGE features. Other disorders with overlapping phenotypes include **cat eye syndrome,** VATER association, and a number of chromosomal syndromes, including trisomy 13, and del (4p) (**Wolf-Hirschhorn syndrome**).

Christian Syndrome

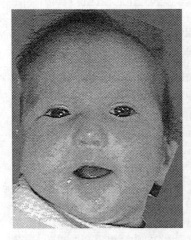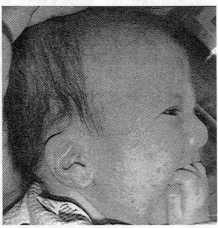

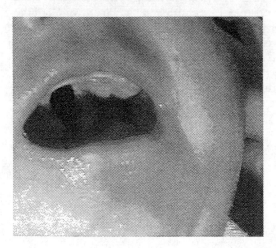

Note micrognathia, low-set posteriorly rotated ears, and U-shaped cleft palate, consistent with Robin sequence associated with Christian syndrome.

Also Known As: Skeletal dysplasia and mental retardation; mental retardation, skeletal dysplasia, and abducens palsy; adducted thumbs syndrome

Christian syndrome has a low prevalence in the general population because early death is common. Originally thought to be autosomal recessive, Christian syndrome was recently mapped to the long arm of the X chromosome.

Major System(s) Affected: Central nervous system; growth; respiratory; skeletal; craniofacial; gastrointestinal; endocrine.

Etiology: X-linked recessive mode of inheritance. The gene has been mapped to Xq28.

Speech Disorders: Speech development has not been observed in patients with Christian syndrome, in part because of severe mental deficiency and in part because of early death.

Feeding Disorders: Early failure-to-thrive should be expected secondary to the combined effects of severe cognitive deficiency, hypotonia, micrognathia, cleft palate, and respiratory compromise (both obstructive and central). Feeding has been difficult, and pneumonias have been reported which may be related to aspiration.

Hearing Disorders: Hearing has not been assessed in children with Christian syndrome.

Voice Disorders: Voice disorders have not been observed or reported in Christian syndrome.

Resonance Disorders: Although cleft palate and hypotonia are both features of the syndrome, because speech does not develop, there have not been opportunities to observe resonance imbalance in speech.

Language Disorders: There is essentially no language development.

Other Clinical Features:

> **Central nervous system:** severe cognitive deficiency; hypotonia; seizures; demyelination of the brain and spinal cord;
>
> **Growth:** growth deficiency;

Respiratory: upper airway obstruction; laryngomalacia; lower respiratory infections; aspiration pneumonia; apnea;

Skeletal: talipes equinovarus; scoliosis; hypoplasia of the sacrum; fusion of cervical vertebrae; thoracic hemivertebrae; pectus excavatum; limitation of extension at the elbows and knees; adducted thumbs;

Craniofacial: micrognathia; Robin sequence; posteriorly rotated ears; metopic ridging; broad nasal root; downslanting eyes; cleft palate; microcephaly;

Gastrointestinal: imperforate anus;

Endocrine: glucose intolerance;

Other: hirsutism.

Natural History: Developmental impairment is obvious from birth, but cognitive impairment worsens with time and the clinical course deteriorates, ending in early death.

Treatment Prognosis: Poor.

Differential Diagnosis: Joint contractures, respiratory compromise, and cleft palate are seen in **distal arthrogryposis syndrome** and in **Freeman-Sheldon syndrome,** but without the severe cognitive impairment seen in Christian syndrome.

Cleidocranial Dysplasia

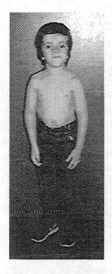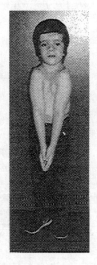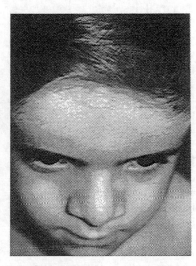

Absence of the clavicles in a 5-year-old boy with cleidocranial dysplasia permitting him to adduct his shoulders. Note the broad forehead (right).

Also Known As: Cleidocranial dysostosis

Cleidocranial dysplasia is a distinctive syndrome that causes unique craniofacial and skeletal abnormalities. These abnormalities make the diagnosis easy to establish in cases that have obvious expressions of the disorder. The population prevalence of the syndrome is not known, but hundreds of cases have been described in the medical literature.

Major System(s) Affected: Craniofacial; dental; skeletal; growth, limbs.

Etiology: Autosomal dominant mode of inheritance. The cause of the disorder is thought to be a deletion at 6p21.

Speech Disorders: Articulation disorders are common in cleidocranial dysplasia. In some cases, there are compensatory substitutions secondary to cleft palate and velopharyngeal insufficiency. However, in the majority of cases, the articulation disorder is related to dental spacing, malocclusions, and missing teeth. The errors are obligatory in nature.

Feeding Disorders: Feeding disorders are not common in cleidocranial dysplasia. Cleft palate is an infrequent finding in the syndrome but can complicate early attempts at feeding. In later life, delayed eruption of the primary and secondary teeth is common and can cause some problems with masticating certain types of food.

Hearing Disorders: Conductive hearing loss is a common finding, caused by minor anomalies of the ossicles and mastoid bone.

Voice Disorders: Voice is typically normal in cleidocranial dysplasia.

Resonance Disorders: Resonance may be hypernasal in cases with cleft palate, but is otherwise normal.

Language Disorders: Language and cognitive development are typically normal.

Other Clinical Features:

Craniofacial: broad forehead, often with bilateral prominence of the frontal bone related to a patent metopic suture; macrocephaly, brachycephaly; late closure of the cranial sutures; large foramen magnum; occasional cleft palate; occasional mild hypertelorism; Class III malocclusion (relative prognathism);

Dental: delayed eruption of both the primary and secondary teeth; over-retained primary dentition with root resporbtion; supernumerary secondary teeth;

Skeletal: absent or hypoplastic clavicles; narrow chest; short ribs; spina bifida occulta; reduced pelvic diameter;

Growth: relatively short stature;

Limbs: brachydactyly, joint laxity.

Natural History: At birth, unless the absence of the clavicles is obvious, the diagnosis can be difficult and the babies look relatively normal. As the cranium and brain begin to grow, the delayed ossification of the cranium and resulting widely patent cranial sutures causes significant distortion of the skull. The head is large, the forehead tall, sometimes with bilateral prominences. The sutures eventually close. Some clinicians have suggested that children with cleidocranial dysplasia wear helmets to protect their brains from injury, but there have not been documented cases of brain trauma related to delayed ossification, possibly because the sutures do have a fibrous connection. As ossification of the cranium occurs, skull shape becomes more normal. Delayed dental eruption is particularly noticeable in the secondary dentition because the primary teeth are often over-retained so that the teeth appear very small and there is severe dental spacing. In females, the reduced pelvic diameter makes normal childbirth difficult so that Caesarean section is necessary.

Treatment Prognosis: The anomalies in cleidocranial dysplasia are not particularly debilitating. Absence of the clavicles does not cause any particular problems and the cranial anomalies resolve with time.

Differential Diagnosis: The association of cranial and clavicular anomalies in cleidocranial dysplasia is essentially unique.

Clouston Syndrome

Also Known As: Hidrotic ectodermal dysplasia; ectodermal dysplasia 2, hydrotic

Clouston syndrome is a rare form of ectodermal dysplasia with normal sweating and cognitive impairment. Other forms of ectodermal dysplasia have deficient sweat and sebaceous glands. Similar to other forms of ectodermal dysplasia, individuals with Clouston syndrome have alopecia, hypoplastic finger- and toenails, but have normal dentition.

Major System(s) Affected: Integument; central nervous system; limbs; ocular.

Etiology: Autosomal dominant mode of inheritance. The gene has been mapped to 13q11-q12.1.

Speech Disorders: Speech is typically delayed and may express neurologically based impairment depending on the severity of cognitive impairment.

Feeding Disorders: Feeding disorders have not been reported or observed.

Hearing Disorders: Hearing loss is not a feature of Clouston syndrome.

Voice Disorders: Voice is normal.

Resonance Disorders: Resonance is typically normal.

Language Disorders: Language impairment is essentially a constant finding and ranges in severity depending on the degree of cognitive impairment. Cognitive disorders range from mild to severe.

Other Clinical Features:

Integument: alopecia varying from sparse hair to total baldness; dysplastic nails; palmar and plantar hyperkeratosis; hyperpigmentation of the skin;

Central nervous system: mental retardation and developmental delay;

Limbs: clubbing of the fingers;

Ocular: strabismus.

Natural History: Because infants often have little hair at birth, and nails are small, the diagnosis of Clouston syndrome can be initially difficult. The hyperkeratosis becomes more prominent with age. Developmental delay is evident early in infancy in many cases.

Treatment Prognosis: The language and speech impairment in Clouston sydrome is static and therefore should repond to aggressive therapy within the limits of the cognitive deficiency.

Differential Diagnosis: There are a number of autosomal dominant forms of ectodermal dysplasia, including **AEC syndrome, Rapp-Hodgkin syndrome,** and **EEC syndrome.** Cognition is typically normal in these syndromes and, unlike Clouston syndrome, the dentition is affected.

Cockayne Syndrome

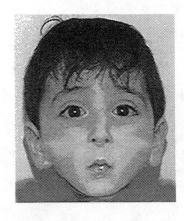

Cockayne syndrome: Note the triangular face with lack of subcutaneous fat in the cheeks.

Also Known As: Cockayne syndrome, type I; Cockayne syndrome, type A

Cockayne syndrome is a rare but distinctive syndrome of premature senility, early death, short stature, and deterioration of the central nervous system. Since its delineation, several subtypes have been identified with different genetic etiologies than the originally described phenotype. The "classic" Cockayne syndrome is now referred to as type I, or type A, by some clinicians.

Major System(s) Affected: Central nervous system; growth; skin; craniofacial; ocular; skeletal; cardiopulmonary, auditory; vascular.

Etiology: Autosomal recessive inheritance.

Speech Disorders: Early speech development and production is often normal through the toddler years. Then speech begins to deteriorate, and dysarthria is a common symptom. Eventually, speech deteriorates to the point of unintelligibility.

Feeding Disorders: Early feeding is normal. When neurologic deterioration begins, feeding may become disordered in a manner similar to that seen in geriatric patients.

Hearing Disorders: Hearing is initially normal, but with the onset of neurologic deterioration, there is perceptual (central) hearing impairment.

Voice Disorders: Voice is high pitched.

Resonance Disorders: Resonance is initially normal, but with the onset of dysarthria, hypernasality may become pronounced.

Language Disorders: Language development is normal in its earliest stages, but during childhood, there is deterioration of all cognitive skills, including language.

Other Clinical Features:

Central nervous system: progressive cognitive impairment; dementia; demyelination;

Growth: short stature;

Skin: photosensitivity; premature aging; pigmentary changes;

Craniofacial: microcephaly; deep-set eyes; relative prognathism;

Ocular: retinal degeneration; retinal pigmentation anomalies; corneal degeneration;

Skeletal: limbs are disproportionately long; large hands and feet; joint contractures;

Cardiopulmonary: hypertension;

Auditory: central deafness;

Vascular: progressive atherosclerosis.

Natural History: Early development after birth may seem relatively normal until 1 to 2 years of age. Progressive cerebellar ataxia, choreoathetosis, and eventually blindness are inevitable and early death occurs following the precipitously downhill neurologic course.

Treatment Prognosis: Poor.

Differential Diagnosis: Premature senility is a key feature of progeria, but without the same neurologic sequelae. Bloom syndrome has similar degenerative skin findings. Progressive neurologic, skin, and visual impairment occur in Refsum syndrome, but without the growth abnormality.

Cockayne Syndrome, Type II

Also Known As: Cockayne syndrome, type B

Cockayne syndrome, type II, is differentiated from type I by the age of onset and progression. The symptoms in Cockayne syndrome, type II, are similar to those of type I, but the expression of the syndrome is congenital, rather than an onset at 2 to 4 years of age as is seen in type I. Individuals with Cockayne syndrome, type II are of low birth weight and grow very little, remaining very small and severely impaired. Although familial cases have not occurred, the gene is expressed in an autosomal dominant manner (i.e., only one mutant copy of the gene pair is required to express the syndrome).

Major System(s) Affected: Central nervous system; growth; skin.

Etiology: Autosomal dominant expression. The gene, ERCC6, has been mapped to 10q11.

Speech Disorders: Speech does not develop.

Feeding Disorders: Feeding is severely impaired by neurologic degeneration. However, very poor growth is a primary feature of the syndrome and is not related to nutrition.

Hearing Disorders: Central hearing impairment is presumed.

Voice Disorders: Voicing for communication does not develop.

Resonance Disorders: Speech does not develop.

Language Disorders: There is no language development.

Other Clinical Features:

> **Central nervous system:** severe mental retardation with progressive degeneration of neurologic function;
>
> **Growth:** very small stature;
>
> **Skin:** hypersensitivity to ultraviolet light.

Natural History: The syndrome is evident at birth and the neurologic findings worsen with age. Premature death is the rule following the progression of early-onset senility.

Treatment Prognosis: Poor.

Differential Diagnosis: The neurologic findings are similar to those in Cockayne syndrome, type I and type III except that the disorder is obvious at birth. **Bloom syndrome** has similar skin findings without the neurological findings.

Cockayne Syndrome, Type III

Also Known As: Cockayne syndrome, type C

Cockayne syndrome, type III, is marked by later onset and slower progression than in types I and II. Older patients have been described who are of normal stature.

Major System(s) Affected: Central nervous system; skin; growth; craniofacial; ocular; skeletal; cardiopulmonary.

Etiology: Autosomal recessive inheritance. The gene has not been mapped or identified.

Speech Disorders: Early speech development is often normal with subsequent deterioration after the onset of neurologic degeneration.

Feeding Disorders: Early feeding is normal. Dysphagia develops following the onset of neurologic deterioration.

Hearing Disorders: Perceptual and sensorineural hearing loss.

Voice Disorders: Voice is normal.

Resonance Disorders: Resonance is normal, but hypernasality may present following the onset of neurologic degeneration.

Language Disorders: Early language development is normal, but deterioration occurs in childhood and adolescence in most cases.

Other Clinical Features:

Central nervous system: neurologic deterioration; mental retardation; early dementia;

Skin: sensitivity to sunlight; pigmentary anomalies; depletion of subcutaneous fat;

Growth: small stature in most cases;

Craniofacial: deep-set eyes; microcephaly; relative prognathism;

Ocular: retinal degeneration; optic atrophy; retinal pigmentation anomalies; corneal degeneration;

Skeletal: long limbs; comparatively large hands and feet;

Cardiopulmonary: hypertension.

Natural History: The progression is the same as type I, but the onset is slightly later and the progression less precipitous. However, the end-stage disease is similar.

Treatment Prognosis: Poor.

Differential Diagnosis: The phenotype is very similar to **Cockayne syndrome, type I.** The skin findings are similar to those seen in **Bloom syndrome.**

Coffin-Lowry Syndrome

Also Known As:

Coffin-Lowry syndrome was initially described in 1966 as a syndrome of severe mental retardation affecting only males. Subsequent observations of less severe manifestations of the disorder in female relatives suggested X-linked dominant expression.

Major System(s) Affected:
Central nervous system; craniofacial; growth; skeletal; cardiac; renal; gastrointestinal; pulmonary.

Etiology: X-linked dominant mode of expression and inheritance. The gene has been mapped to Xp22.2-p22.1.

Speech Disorders: Affected males do not develop speech because of severe mental retardation.

Feeding Disorders: Early hypotonia may impair feeding and cause failure-to-thrive.

Hearing Disorders: Sensorineural hearing loss has been observed in some cases, ranging from moderate to severe.

Voice Disorders: Voice is not used for speech in affected males, but hoarseness during vocalizations is common.

Resonance Disorders: Resonance disorders have not been observed primarily because of the lack of speech development in affected males.

Language Disorders: Language is severely impaired, usually to the point of absence of language development in males. Female heterozygotes have mild to moderate language impairment.

Other Clinical Features:

Central nervous system: mental retardation, typically severe in males; hypotonia; hydrocephalus;

Craniofacial: coarse facial appearance; broad, flat nose; thick lips; anteverted nostrils; large ears; telecanthus; large mouth; prominent supraorbital ridge;

Growth: short stature; postnatal growth deficiency;

Musculoskeletal: cervical lordosis; kyphoscoliosis; pectus carinatum; flat feet; hyperextensible joints; tapered digits;

Cardiac: mitral valve regurgitation;

Renal: hydronephrosis;

Gastrointestinal: diverticulosis;

Pulmonary: restrictive pulmonary disease.

Natural History: Growth deficiency is of postnatal onset. Developmental impairment is evident very early. Postural changes, possibly secondary to hypotonia, lead to scoliosis, kyphosis, and cervical lordosis.

Treatment Prognosis: Very poor in males. Female heterozygotes typically have cognitive development ranging from normal to mildly impaired, although some are severely impaired.

Differential Diagnosis: The early facial appearance and hypotonia are somewhat reminiscent of **Williams syndrome,** but the absence of speech and language development soon differentiate the two diagnoses. The coarse facial features may also be mistaken for lysosomal storage diseases that can be ruled out by metabolic testing.

Coffin-Siris Syndrome

Also Known As: Fifth digit syndrome

This autosomal dominant syndrome of mental retardation is one of a number of multiple anomaly syndromes associated with Dandy-Walker anomaly, a cystlike malformation of the brain involving enlargement of the fourth ventricle, hypoplasia/aplasia of the cerebellar vermis, and posterior fossa cyst. A distinctive feature of the syndrome is absence of the nails on the fifth fingers and toes. Feeding and speech disorders are typically severe. There is a 4:1 ratio of affected females to males, suggesting lethality in at least some males.

Major System(s) Affected: Central nervous system; growth; craniofacial; limbs; hair.

Etiology: Autosomal dominant mode of expression. The gene has not been mapped or identified.

Speech Disorders: Few patients with Coffin-Siris syndrome develop speech, even if their language comprehension is good. The absence of speech development is sometimes disproportionate to the degree of cognitive deficiency.

Feeding Disorders: Feeding is often severely impaired in infancy from a combination of hypotonia and respiratory compromise. Failure-to-thrive is the rule rather than the exception in Coffin-Siris syndrome.

Hearing Disorders: Hearing loss has not been documented or observed as a feature of Coffin-Siris syndrome.

Voice Disorders: Wet hoarseness during crying is common and related to chronic upper and lower respiratory illness.

Resonance Disorders: Resonance disorders have not been reported or observed.

Language Disorders: Receptive language impairment is variable, ranging from normal to severely impaired, but expressive language is essentially always impaired, usually severely.

Other Clinical Features:

Central nervous system: cognitive impairment; severe hypotonia; seizures; Dandy-Walker malformation;

Growth: prenatal growth deficiency;

Craniofacial: coarse facial appearance; thick lips; microcephaly; ptosis; broad nose; choanal atresia or stenosis;

Limbs: absence of the nails on the fifth fingers and toes; absent distal phalanges of the fifth toes; small patellae;

Hair: sparse scalp hair.

Natural History: The syndrome manifests at birth with low birth weight and early feeding and respiratory difficulties. Failure-to-thrive is common and is complicated by hypotonia. Motor milestones are all delayed, but expressive language is more impaired than other developmental landmarks.

Treatment Prognosis: The prognosis for speech therapy is poor.

Differential Diagnosis: The coarse facial features are somewhat similar to **Coffin-Lowry syndrome,** but the sparse scalp hair soon differentiates the two disorders.

Cohen Syndrome

Also Known As: Pepper syndrome

First described in 1973 as a syndrome of obesity, hypotonia, and cognitive impairment, this autosomal recessive disorder is probably under-reported and more common than previously suspected. The pattern, while distinctive, is not associated with severely dysmorphic features.

Major System(s) Affected: Central nervous system; growth; craniofacial; limbs; cardiac; hematologic; ocular.

Etiology: Autosomal recessive mode of inheritance. The gene has been mapped to 8q22-q23 and has been labelled COH1.

Speech Disorders: Speech is often delayed in onset and articulation may be slow and deliberate in childhood. Hypotonia tends to affect rate, which is slower than normal, especially in patients with more severe cognitive impairment. Articulation is marked by anterior distortions related to malocclusion (maxillary overbite).

Feeding Disorders: Hypotonia may cause poor sucking in infancy, thus prolonging early feeding, but failure-to-thrive is not associated with Cohen syndrome.

Hearing Disorders: Hearing loss is not a feature of Cohen syndrome.

Voice Disorders: Voice disorders have not been documented or observed in patients with Cohen syndrome.

Resonance Disorders: There is often a muffled oral resonance, and occasional mixed hyper-hyponasality which may be indicative of a mild dysarthria.

Language Disorders: Language onset is almost always delayed, usually mildly. Language impairment is commensurate with degree of cognitive impairment. Length of utterance is often reduced.

Other Clinical Features:

   Central nervous system: cognitive impairment, usually mild; hypotonia; seizures;

Growth: obesity; short stature; delayed onset of puberty;

Craniofacial: vertical maxillary excess; "high arched" palate; retruded mandible, prominent maxillary central incisors; downslanting eyes; prominent nasal root;

Limbs: hyperextensible joints; thin fingers; narrow hands and small feet;

Cardiac: mitral valve prolapse; ventriculoseptal defect;

Hematologic: leukopenia;

Ocular: iris and retina coloboma; chorioretinopathy; macular anomalies.

Natural History: Birth weight tends to be low. The onset of obesity is in childhood. Hypotonia persists from birth into adult life. There is delayed sexual maturation.

Treatment Prognosis: The prognosis for improvement in speech and language is good for those patients with mild cognitive impairment, which is the majority of patients with Cohen syndrome. However, in the small percentage of cases with more severe cognitive impairment, the prognosis for improvement is reduced.

Differential Diagnosis: Although there are other syndromes associated with hypotonia and obesity, such as **Prader-Willi syndrome**, the **Bardet-Biedl syndromes**, **Laurence-Moon syndrome**, the pattern of anomalies in Cohen syndrome is distinctive and is not marked by hyperphagia (as in **Prader-Willi syndrome**) or the severe obesity seen in the **Bardet-Biedl syndromes**.

Cowden Syndrome

Also Known As: Cowden disease; multiple hamartoma syndrome

Cowden syndrome is a disorder that causes hamartomas, nodular neoplasias, in multiple areas of the body including the lips, tongue, oral gingiva, and palate. Hamartomatous growths also occur in glandular tissue, including the thyroid gland and the breasts.

Major System(s) Affected: Central nervous system; endocrine/glandular; skin; skeletal; craniofacial; gastrointestinal.

Etiology: Autosomal dominant inheritance. The gene, a tumor suppressor gene labeled PTEN, has been mapped to 10q23.3.

Speech Disorders: Articulation may be impaired in a number of ways related to the presence of oral hamartomas. Tongue placement can be altered because the surface of the tongue is not flat or smooth enough to make a broad contact with the alveolus, teeth, or palate. The lips may also have difficulty creating a tight seal because of multiple hamartomas. Distortions may also be caused by obligatory redirection of the airstream.

Feeding Disorders: The hamartomas occur later in life, usually in adolescence or early adult life, and are not present at birth. Early feeding is normal, and the hamartomas typically do not interfere with feeding in adult life, unless they require extensive surgical resection. Some of the hamartomas have been reported to develop into carcinomas requiring treatment.

Hearing Disorders: Sensorineural hearing loss is a low frequency anomaly in Cowden syndrome.

Voice Disorders: Hoarseness is a common feature.

Resonance Disorders: Oral resonance may be muffled related to larger neoplasias in the oral cavity, especially posteriorly. Hyponasality may also occur related to adenoid enlargement.

Language Disorders: A small percentage of patients with Cowden syndrome may have mild cognitive impairment causing a language delay. In most cases, language is normal.

Other Clinical Features:

Central nervous system: increased intracranial pressure; cognitive impairment in some cases; seizures; cerebellar anomalies; Chiari anomaly;

Endocrine/glandular: hamartomas of the thyroid and breast;

Skin: multiple hamartomas of the mucous membrane, particularly of the oral cavity; skin lesions on the face and limbs;

Skeletal: pectus excavatum; scoliosis;

Craniofacial: macrencephaly; oral hamartomas;

Gastrointestinal: polypoid growth in the intestines;

Other: potential cancerous neoplasia of the brain, breast, skin, or kidneys.

Natural History: The hamartomas begin to develop in late childhood or early adolescence and become larger and more numerous with age. Many of the neurological symptoms are related to later tumor growth and are not present in early life.

Treatment Prognosis: Symptomatic treatment may be valuable in removing particularly large growths that interfere with speech, but in some cases, the treatment may not improve function because the resection itself may leave excessive scar tissue. Additional growths may also appear in nearby tissues.

Differential Diagnosis: A number of syndromes may cause changes in the skin and mucous membrane of the oral cavity, including acanthosis nigricans, and Gardner syndrome has intestinal polyps. **Proteus syndrome,** the disorder expressed by the Elephant Man, results in many hamartomas, but they occur in regions other than the oral cavity and intestines.

Craniodiaphyseal Dysplasia

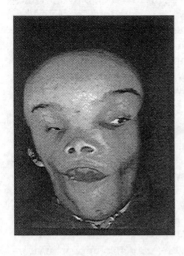

Severe craniofacial overgrowth associated with craniodiaphyseal dysplasia.

Also Known As: Leontiasis

Craniodiaphyseal dysplasia is a rare syndrome of bony overgrowth of the craniofacial structures with associated abnormalities of the long bones. The overgrowth of the craniofacial skeleton is severe and may result in life-threatening compromise of the central nervous system and respiratory tract. The disorder was brought to public attention in the motion picture *Mask*.

Major System(s) Affected: Skeletal; craniofacial; central nervous system.

Etiology: The majority of cases that have been reported are of autosomal recessive etiology. However, autosomal dominant transmission of the syndrome has been observed. A gene has not been mapped or identified.

Speech Disorders: Speech onset may be delayed. Bony overgrowth results in malocclusion and severe crowding of the oral cavity because of hyperostoses on the palate and jaws. Oral opening may be limited. There is severe articulatory impairment because of obligatory placement errors.

Feeding Disorders: In the neonatal period and infancy, feeding is not typically impaired. As the nasal cavity become increasingly more obstructed, there may be some difficulty with eating. Later in life, diet may need to be shifted to soft foods because of severe occlusal anomalies.

Hearing Disorders: Mixed hearing loss is constant beginning in early childhood, related to anomalies of the cranial bones, including the mastoid and ossicles. The hearing loss is typically progressive with eventual maximal or near maximal conductive loss and progressive neural loss related to compression of the cranial nerves.

Voice Disorders: Voice disorders have not been reported or observed.

Resonance Disorders: Resonance becomes progressively more hyponasal with age, beginning in childhood. By adult life, there is total denasality. Oral resonance is also disordered because of maxillary and palatal skeletal overgrowth.

Language Disorders: Language may be normal in early life, although in some cases, there has been marked delay, especially of expressive language. With age and progressive compression of the brain, additional language impairment and cognitive impairment may occur.

Other Clinical Features:

Skeletal: diaphyseal dysplasia; absence of metaphyseal flaring of the long bones; sclerosis of mutliple skeletal components;

Craniofacial: severe overgrowth of the craniofacial skeleton leading to compromise of the nasal cavity, constriction of the cranial foramina, and compression of multiple nerves and blood vessels; orbital hypertelorism;

Central nervous system: compression of the cranial nerves; occasional cognitive impairment; increased intracranial pressure.

Natural History: The disorder is expressed shortly after birth and becomes obvious in childhood. The skeletal overgrowth reaches severe proportions quickly and compression of the cranial nerves becomes evident by the second decade of life. Respiratory obstruction also becomes progressively worse with severe obstructive sleep apnea caused by progressive narrowing of the upper airway because of skeletal overgrowth. The foramen magnum and other cranial foramina and fossae become obliterated or constricted and may result in sensory hearing loss, blindness, and early death. Increased intracranial pressure may result in progressive cognitive impairment. Obliteration of the sella turcica and pituitary gland results in lack of sexual maturation and short stature.

Treatment Prognosis: Poor. The disorder is relentlessly progressive and palliative treatments will have only temporary benefit.

Differential Diagnosis: Skeletal overgrowth of the craniofacial complex is common in **van Buchem disease,** osteosclerosis, **craniometaphyseal dysplasia,** and **frontometaphyseal dysplasia.** Craniodiaphyseal dysplasia differs from these other disorders in relation to the appearance of the long bones, which have absence of metaphyseal flaring.

Craniofrontonasal Syndrome

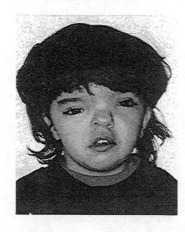

Craniofrontonasal dysplasia syndrome: Note severe hypertelorism and orbital asymmetry.

Also Known As: Craniofrontonasal dysplasia; craniofrontonasal dysostosis

This X-linked syndrome results in a wide variety of craniofacial anomalies, including orbital hypertelorism, orbital dystopia, cleft palate, or cleft lip and palate. Hypertelorism is typically severe.

Major System(s) Affected: Craniofacial; integument; limbs; skeletal; genital; central nervous system.

Etiology: The disorder is inherited in an X-linked manner, but the mechanism of expression does not fit either dominant or recessive patterns. Inconsistent with X-linked dominant inheritance is the observation that the majority of familial cases observed and reported have been female-to-female transmission. The majority of known cases have been female, leading to initial speculation of male lethality of a possible X-linked dominant trait. However, several male cases have been reported that are more mildly affected than females, an observation that is inconsistent with X-linked dominant transmission. However, no male-to-male cases have been observed, indicative that the gene is on the X chromosome. The gene has been mapped to Xp22.

Speech Disorders: Speech production is often affected by occlusal abnormalities resulting in obligatory distortions and substitutions. The presence of cleft palate or cleft lip and palate may result in compensatory articulation patterns.

Feeding Disorders: Feeding in infancy may be complicated by cleft palate, but is otherwise not impaired.

Hearing Disorders: Conductive hearing loss secondary to chronic middle ear effusion is common.

Voice Disorders: Hoarseness has been observed in some cases.

Resonance Disorders: Hypernasality secondary to cleft palate is common.

Language Disorders: Language impairment has been observed, as has cognitive impairment in some cases. However, language is often normal.

Other Clinical Features:

> **Craniofacial:** orbital hypertelorism; orbital dystopia; cleft lip; cleft palate; low set posteriorly rotated ears; broad nose with bifid tip;

> **Integument:** coarse, wiry hair; longitudinal splitting of the fingernails;

> **Skeletal:** Sprengel shoulder; pectus excavatum; clavicle anomalies;

> **Genital:** hypospadias in males;

> **Central nervous system:** occasional mental retardation; absence of the corpus callosum; learning disabilities.

Natural History: The disorder presents at birth and is not progressive.

Treatment Prognosis: Reconstructive surgery is indicated for resolution of structural anomalies. The prognosis with current craniofacial surgery techniques is good.

Differential Diagnosis: Orbital hypertelorism or craniofacial anomalies in association with clavicle anomalies is seen in **cleidocranial dysplasia.** Isolated frontonasal dysplasia has very similar facial features, but no associated anomalies.

Craniometaphyseal Dysplasia

Also Known As:

Craniometaphyseal dysplasia occurs in two forms that are etiologically distinct, but clinically identical. The syndrome is marked by overgrowth of the craniofacial skeleton and generalized skeletal sclerosis and dysplasia of the long bones. Both the dominant and recessive forms are rare disorders.

Major System(s) Affected:
Craniofacial; skeletal; central nervous system.

Etiology:
An autosomal dominant form has been mapped to 5p15.2-p14.1. The recessive form has not been mapped, nor the gene identified.

Speech Disorders:
Obligatory articulation disorders include distortions secondary to malocclusion and anterior skeletal open-bite. The open-bite is caused by chronic open-mouth posture related to nasal obstruction from skeletal overgrowth. Eventually, cranial nerve compression may result in facial paresis and poor mobility of the oral musculature resulting in dysarthric speech production.

Feeding Disorders:
Feeding is normal in infancy. After the beginning of craniofacial osteosclerosis, nasal obstruction ensues causing chronic mouth-breathing and some difficulty with large amounts of food being maintained in the mouth.

Hearing Disorders:
Progressive mixed hearing loss is common and is related to sclerosis of the temporal bone and mastoids. Hearing loss begins in childhood and progresses to severe levels later in adult life.

Voice Disorders:
Voice disorders have not been reported.

Resonance Disorders:
Resonance is hyponasal related to bony stenosis of the nasal cavity.

Language Disorders:
Language development is normal.

Other Clinical Features:

Craniofacial: skeletal dysplasia and sclerosis; orbital hypertelorism; nasal stenosis; broad nasal root; facial paresis;

Skeletal: metaphyseal dysplasia; metaphyseal flaring;

Central nervous system: possible blindness secondary to optic nerve compression; occasional cognitive impairment.

Natural History: The onset of observable structural change in the face begins in late infancy or toddler years, usually with marked broadening of the nasal root. Progressive sclerosis proceeds unabated into adult life with resulting compression of cranial nerves II, VII, and VIII.

Treatment Prognosis: Palliative treatment has only temporary effects because the bone growth continues throughout life.

Differential Diagnosis: There are a number of syndromes with progressive sclerotic growth of bone, including **van Buchem syndrome,** sclerosteosis, Pyle disease, **craniodiapheseal dysplasia,** and **frontometaphyseal dysplasia.** The differential diagnosis is based on radiographic differences in the type of skeletal dysplasia and the bones affected.

Cri-du-Chat Syndrome

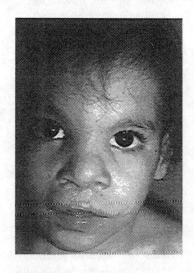

Infant with bilateral cleft lip and palate secondary to cri-du-chat syndrome (del 5p).

Also Known As: Cat cry syndrome; del(5p) syndrome

Cri-du-chat syndrome is distinctive in relation to the high-pitched cry in the neonatal period and infancy that resembles the mewing of a cat. Although the cry is distinctive, it is not a constant feature in the syndrome and does not appear to be related to structural anomalies of the larynx. The specific mechanism of the cry is, as yet, unknown. The syndrome has an estimated population prevalence of 1:50,000.

Major System(s) Affected: Central nervous system; growth; craniofacial; gastrointestinal; musculoskeletal.

Etiology: Deletion of a portion of the short arm of chromosome 5, specifically 5p15.2. The size of the deletion has been variable in reported cases, ranging from only band 5p12.2 to the entire short arm of chromosome 5.

Speech Disorders: The majority of individuals with cri-du-chat do not develop speech. Although

135

the degree of cognitive impairment is variable, essentially all cases have severe retardation. Communication is further impaired in cases that have cleft palate or cleft lip and palate.

Feeding Disorders: Early failure-to-thrive occurs in many cases related to severe neurological deficits and hypotonia. Cleft palate or cleft lip and palate may further complicate early feeding.

Hearing Disorders: Conductive hearing loss secondary to chronic middle ear effusion is common.

Voice Disorders: The high-pitched cry that is characteristic in many patients with cri-du-chat persists throughout infancy, but true voice is rarely used for communication.

Resonance Disorders: Speech is typically not developed so that resonance balance is not an issue.

Language Disorders: Language development is typically absent or very severely impaired.

Other Clinical Features:

Central nervous system: severe cognitive impairment; cerebral asymmetry; early hypotonia followed by hypertonia and hyperreflexia;

Growth: small stature;

Craniofacial: microcephaly; retrognathia; craniofacial asymmetry; relative hypertelorism; cleft palate or cleft lip and palate; Robin sequence; prominent nasal root; low-set posteriorly rotated ears;

Gastrointestinal: malrotation of the bowel; megacolon;

Musculoskeletal: joint contractures; small hands and feet; talipes equinovarus.

Natural History: Failure-to-thrive and respiratory compromise are common in infancy. Many infants do not survive the newborn period. Life span in general is decreased.

Treatment Prognosis: Poor.

Differential Diagnosis: The diagnosis is easily confirmed by karyotype.

Crouzon Syndrome

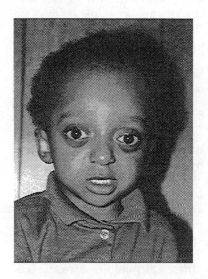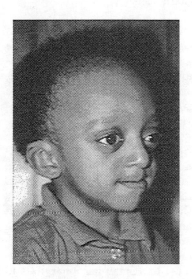

Four-year-old boy with Crouzon syndrome. Note the exorbitism and maxillary deficiency.

Also Known As: Craniofacial dysostosis

Crouzon syndrome has been recognized as a genetic syndrome since its publication by Crouzon in 1912. In the past, many disorders with craniosynostosis were given the diagnostic label of Crouzon sydrome, probably inappropriately. Many new syndromes of craniosynostosis have been described since the delineation of Crouzon, and it is likely that many cases of **Pfeiffer syndrome, Jackson-Weiss syndrome,** and others have been mistakenly lumped together with Crouzon. The population prevalence of Crouzon syndrome is probably near 1:25,000 people. Crouzon differs from other syndromes of craniosynostosis in that all of the findings are limited to the craniofacial skeleton.

Major System(s) Affected: Craniofacial.

Etiology: Crouzon syndrome is caused by mutation of a single gene, FGFR2 (fibroblast growth factor receptor 2) located on the long arm of chromosome 10. Inheritance is autosomal dominant with variable expression.

Speech Disorders: Articulation disorders are very common, marked by obligatory distortions related to malocclusion, especially Class III maxillary retrusions and anterior skeletal open-bites, which are common in the syndrome. Resonance may also be hyponasal related to a small nasopharynx and nasal cavity. Cleft palate is a rare finding in the syndrome and is unlikely to cause significant hypernasality because of the reduced size of the nasopharynx.

Feeding Disorders: Upper airway obstruction and possible choanal atresia will result in failure-to-thrive because infants with Crouzon syndrome will strive to maintain respiration even at the expense of feeding. In such cases, the airway obstruction must be relieved.

Hearing Disorders: Conductive hearing loss is common, usually mild, occasionally moderate, related to chronic middle ear disease, chronic fluid, ossicular anomalies, or any combination of the three.

Voice Disorders: Not a component of this syndrome.

Resonance Disorders: Hyponasality is common related to reduced nasal cavity size and reduced nasopharyngeal volume.

Language Disorders: Language development is usually normal, unless there are sequelae of increased intracranial pressure.

Other Clinical Features: Maxillary hypoplasia, Class III malocclusion, occasional soft tissue hypertrophy of the hard palate, occasional cognitive impairment secondary to increased intracranial pressure and resulting brain damage, conductive hearing loss is common caused by both synostoses of the ossicles, and by reduced eustachian tube function. Eustachian tube dysfunction is related to two factors: abnormal skull configuration caused by the craniosynostosis results in an abnormal angulation and diameter of the tube; and the middle ear space is reduced in size, and therefore, is more easily filled with fluid. The clinical features of Crouzon syndrome are essentially limited to the craniofacial complex and the consequences of cranio-synostosis. Abnormal skull shape, exorbitism (bulging eyes), maloc-clusion, dental crowding, ocular papilladema, and abnormal angu-lation of the ears are all secondary to the deforming effects of the skel-etal growth abnormality of the cra-nial and facial bones. Hydroce-phalus may occur, although less frequently than in **Apert syndrome** and **Pfeiffer syndrome.** Cleft pal-ate has been reported in a small number of cases. Other findings, es-pecially extracranial anomalies, are very rare and may be coincidental.

Natural History: Many infants with Crouzon syndrome appear normal at birth, although in some cases, the effects of synostosis are already apparent. With growth and age, progressive worsening of the midface deficiency becomes evi-dent, becoming most obvious with the 6th year and pubertal growth spurts. If there is increasing intra-cranial pressure, there may be some neurologic deterioration, preceded by headaches, ataxia, or other psy-chomotor symptoms. The majority of patients with Crouzon syn-drome have normal intellect and

development if the craniosynosto-sis is surgically corrected early in life (the optimal time being in infancy).

Treatment Prognosis: The prognosis for normal cognitive de-velopment is excellent, especially if craniectomy or cranial reconstruc-tion is accomplished early in life. Children with Crouzon syndrome should be continuously checked for increased intracranial pressure un-til brain growth is complete. Oblig-atory articulation errors are related to skeletal anomalies that cause maloclusions. Therefore, resolution of the anterior sound distortions in Crouzon syndrome would not be expected until after correction of the occlusal anomalies by ortho-gnathic surgery or mid-face ad-vancement.

Differential Diagnosis: There are a number of syndromes that have craniosynostosis as a primary finding, including **Apert** and **Jack-son-Weiss syndromes,** which are caused by a different mutation in the same FGFR2 gene that causes Crouzon syndrome. Crouzon syn-drome may be distinguished from other syndromes of craniosynosto-sis by the absence of limb anomalies and the better cognitive prognosis.

Cryptophthalmos Syndrome

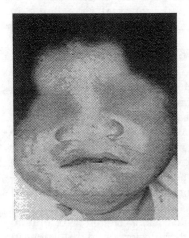

Cryptophthalmos syndrome: Note the absence of palpebral openings and the extension of hair onto the lateral aspects of the forehead.

Also Known As: Fraser syndrome; cryptophthalmos-syndactyly syndrome

This distinctive syndrome involves cryptophthalmos (meaning "hidden eyes"). The syndrome's identifying characteristic is absence of palpebral fissures, but the eyes may be normal underneath a skin covering in some cases.

Major System(s) Affected: Ocular; craniofacial; limbs; gastrointestinal; genitourinary; central nervous system.

Etiology: Autosomal recessive inheritance. The gene has not been mapped or identified.

Speech Disorders: Speech is delayed in most cases secondary to cognitive impairment. Articulation may also be impaired by compensatory articulation patterns in cases with cleft palate or cleft lip and palate (approximately 10%).

Feeding Disorders: Infant feeding may be compromised by respiratory distress secondary to laryngeal stenosis. Cleft palate may further complicate feeding.

Hearing Disorders: Conductive hearing loss secondary to ossicular malformations is common. The external ear canal may also be stenotic.

Voice Disorders: Voice disorders have not been reported or observed.

Resonance Disorders: Hypernasal resonance may occur in patients with cleft palate.

Language Disorders: Language delay and impairment are common because of the frequency of cognitive impairment in the syndrome.

Other Clinical Features:

Ocular: cryptophthalmos; eyelid coloboma; dermoid cysts; absent lens; corneal opacity; absent lacrimal glands;

Craniofacial: craniofacial asymmetry; hypertelorism; auricular anomalies; low set ears; stenotic external auditory meatus; cleft palate plus/minus cleft lip; bifid nose or nasal tip; low anterior hairline; projection of hair on the face near the eyes;

Limbs: syndactyly;

Gastrointestinal: umbilical hernia; omphalocele; abnormal placement of umbilicus;

Genitourinary: renal anomalies; clitoral enlargement; malformed fallopian tubes; bicornate uterus; small male genitalia; hypospadias; cryptorchidism;

Central nervous system: cognitive impairment; encephalocele; Dandy-Walker anomaly.

Natural History: Some affected infants are stillborn or die shortly after birth. Blindness is typical, but sight has been restored by surgical means in some cases. Ambiguity of the genitalia has been seen and may result in ambiguous gender identity.

Treatment Prognosis: Overall prognosis is dependent on the degree of cognitive impairment.

Differential Diagnosis: There are no syndromes with significant phenotypic overlap with cryptophthalmos syndrome.

De Barsy Syndrome

Also Known As: Cutis laxa with corneal clouding and mental retardation

De Barsy syndrome is a rare syndrome of mental retardation associated with microcephaly, small stature, and loose skin caused by abnormalities in the elastic fibers of the skin.

Major System(s) Affected: Central nervous system; growth; integument; ocular; musculoskeletal.

Etiology: Autosomal recessive inheritance. The gene has not been mapped or identified.

Speech Disorders: Patients with De Barsy syndrome are unlikely to develop significant speech.

Feeding Disorders: Early hypotonia and poor oral coordination are common and may lead to feeding disorders and failure-to-thrive.

Hearing Disorders: Hearing is within normal limits.

Voice Disorders: Voice is often hoarse and there is some redundancy of the mucosa of the vocal cords (author's observation).

Resonance Disorders: There is insufficient speech for assessing resonance, but generalized dysarthria or oral movement is common.

Language Disorders: There is severe language impairment, often with absent development of expressive language.

Other Clinical Features:

Central nervous system: mental retardation; hypotonia; athetosis;

Growth: growth deficiency of prenatal onset; very small stature;

Integument: cutis laxa (loose skin);

Ocular: corneal opacity; cataracts;

Musculoskeletal: hip dislocation; thumb and hallux dislocations.

Natural History: Loose skin is noted at birth, as is hypotonia, and eventually developmental delay. With age, the child looks prematurely old because the skin is wizened. There is global developmental impairment.

Treatment Prognosis: Poor.

Differential Diagnosis: A number of syndromes show evidence of premature aging, including acrogeria, progeria, granddad syndrome, and gerodermia osteodysplastica. However, these syndromes do not have mental retardation as a component.

D

de Lange Syndrome

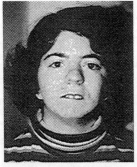 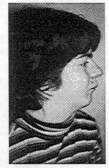

de Lange Syndrome: Facial appearance of an adolescent with de Lange syndrome (above) with minor limb reduction anomalies, including shortening of the fifth fingers bilaterally.

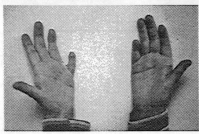 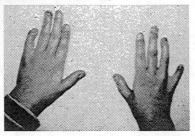

Also Known As: Cornelia de Lange syndrome; Brachmann-de Lange syndrome

de Lange syndrome is a distinctive syndrome of mental retardation and small stature that is easily recognized and one of the more common multiple anomaly disorders associated with severe cognitive impairment. The population prevalence of de Lange syndrome is probably between 1:10,000 and 1:15,000. There is marked variability of expression.

Major System(s) Affected: Central nervous system; growth; limbs; craniofacial; integument; dental; musculoskeletal; cardiac; gastrointestinal; hematologic; genitals.

Etiology: The very large majority of de Lange cases are sporadic, but

144

an autosomal dominant mode of expression and inheritance has been suggested based on a small number of vertical pedigree transmissions. Trisomy of 3q26.3 has been found in a number of cases, but not all, and a single gene responsible for the syndrome located at 3q26.3 is possible, if not likely.

Speech Disorders: A high percentage of patients with de Lange syndrome are severely retarded and do not develop speech at all. However, more mildly affected cases have been recognized, and even though IQ does approach normal values, speech development is more severely impaired than other cognitive skills and the onset of speech is severely delayed. Articulation is frequently impaired by a combination of factors including severe malocclusion problems (micrognathia and Class II malocclusion) and compensatory substitutions related to cleft palate. Retro-micrognathia (the lower jaw is both retruded and small) results in severe tongue backing and articulation impairment.

Feeding Disorders: Early feeding problems are very common in de Lange syndrome with failure-to-thrive a nearly consistent finding. The early feeding disorders are multifactorial in nature, contributed to by upper airway obstruction (micrognathia), dystonia and opisthotonic posture, esophageal stenosis, heart malformations, diaphragmatic hernia, and gastroesophageal reflux.

Hearing Disorders: Hearing loss is probably under-reported in de Lange syndrome, in part because the frequency of severe retardation and early death are so common. Both conductive and sensorineural hearing loss may occur in the syndrome. Conductive loss is secondary to chronic middle ear disease and effusion, sometimes related to cleft palate. Sensorineural hearing loss is variable, from mild to severe, and usually bilateral.

Voice Disorders: Hoarseness is common and may be detected in the early crying of babies with de Lange syndrome. The cry is often low pitched, as well.

Resonance Disorders: Both hypernasality and hyponasality may be observed. Hypernasality is common in the individuals with de Lange syndrome who have cleft palate. Hyponasality may occur in some cases because the nasal capsule is smaller than normal. Abnormal oral resonance is also common because of severe retro-micrognathia that causes the tongue to fall posteriorly in the oropharynx and hypopharynx producing a muffling of oral resonance.

Language Disorders: Language is often more severely impaired than would be expected in relation to the degree of cognitive impairment. In cases with severe cognitive impairment, expressive language rarely develops. In cases with less severe cognitive impairment, expressive language is typically more severely impaired than receptive language, and failure to develop expressive language is observed even in cases with moderate retardation. Because there is often limb reduction and absence of multiple digits in de Lange syndrome, signing may not be possible.

Other Clinical Features:

Central nervous system: mental retardation; hypertonia; opisthotonic posture; seizures;

Growth: small stature; low birth weight;

Limbs: limb reduction (phocomelia); missing digits, shortening of the forearms; absent tibia; bifurcate femur; low set thumbs;

Craniofacial: thin upper lip; downturned oral commissures; retro-micrognathia; low set posteriorly rotated ears; minor external ear anomalies; microcephaly;

Integument: hirsutism; synophrys; arched and flared eyebrows; hair growth on forehead and down the neck; cutis marmorata; multiple deeply pigmented nevi;

Dental: small teeth; dental spacing;

Musculoskeletal: limited joint mobility; delayed skeletal maturation;

Cardiac: heart anomalies (VSD, ASD, hypoplastic left ventricle);

Gastrointestinal: diaphragmatic hernia; esophageal/ pyloric stenosis; duplication of the colon; Meckel's diverticulum; gastroesophageal reflux;

Hematologic: thrombocytopenia;

Genitourinary: hypoplastic kidneys; cryptorchidism and

hypospadias in males; bicornate uterus in females.

Natural History: Developmental milestones are globally delayed, but the onset of speech and language is far more severely impaired and rarely becomes commensurate with overall development. Life expectancy is shortened in many cases. Many infants develop pneumonias and other respiratory disorders with failure-to-thrive, many succumbing in the neonatal period.

Treatment Prognosis: Variable, ranging from fair to poor in many areas, but typically poor in relation to expressive language and speech. A high percentage of individuals with de Lange syndrome are institutionalized.

Differential Diagnosis: The coarse facial appearance associated with mental retardation seen in de Lange syndrome may have some similarities to **Coffin-Siris syndrome.** However, the clinical manifestations of de Lange syndrome are very distinctive and diagnosis is not difficult.

D

Diastrophic Dysplasia

Also Known As: Diastrophic nanism syndrome

Diastrophic dysplasia is a syndrome of short stature and short limbs with craniofacial anomalies. It is one of a small number of syndromes of short stature that leads to the Robin sequence because of the micrognathia caused by the genetic defect.

Major System(s) Affected: Growth; craniofacial; skeletal; limbs.

Etiology: Autosomal recessive inheritance. The gene has been mapped to 5q32-q33.1. The gene has been labelled DTDST for *d*iastrophic *d*ysplasia *s*ulfate *t*ransporter.

Speech Disorders: Articulation may be impaired by malocclusion (micrognathia, sometimes with anterior skeletal open-bite) resulting in lingual protrusion. Articulation may also be impaired by compensatory substitutions secondary to cleft palate and velopharyngeal insufficiency.

Feeding Disorders: Early feeding is often impaired related to upper airway obstruction and possible lower airway disorders related to pulmonary restriction. Robin sequence with micrognathia can contribute to the airway and feeding disorders. Cleft palate may occur, further aggravating attempts to feed. Aspiration has been reported, presumably secondary to negative pressure in the upper airway secondary to glossoptosis. Laryngeal cartilage anomalies may also contribute to airway obstruction.

Hearing Disorders: Conductive hearing loss secondary to middle ear effusion may occur in those cases with cleft palate.

Voice Disorders: Hoarseness is common, and may even be noticeable in the infant cry. Hoarseness may be caused by laryngeal cartilage anomalies (lack of cartilage flexibility with abnormal ossification) and chronic respiratory compromise and congestion.

Resonance Disorders: There are multiple resonance abnormalities in diastrophic dysplasia including nasal resonance and oral resonance disorders. Hypernasality is common secondary to cleft palate, a common clinical feature of the syndrome. Oral resonance is often muffled and damped by micrognathia and a relatively short neck and pharynx.

Language Disorders: Language development is typically normal.

Other Clinical Features:

Growth: disproportionate short stature, short limb variety;

Craniofacial: micrognathia; hypertrophic external ear cartilage; ossification of the auricles; cleft palate; Robin sequence; long philtrum; short nose;

Skeletal: rib cartilage calcification; cervical spine subluxation; kyphoscoliosis; lordosis;

Limbs: abnormal angulation of the thumb ("hitchhiker thumb"); symphalangism; brachydactyly; club foot; short arms and legs.

Natural History: The early neonatal period is difficult for many in-dividuals with diastrophic dysplasia because of potentially severe respiratory complications, feeding difficulty, and failure-to-thrive. The syndrome is marked by progressive ossification of cartilaginous structures, including the lower airway and ribs, thus causing restrictive pulmonary disease. Those individuals who survive the neonatal period and infancy have normal intellectual development. Adult height is averages approximately four feet (125 cm).

Treatment Prognosis: In some cases, the airway restriction is so severe that early treatment fails and death ensues. However, most patients can be managed successfully and will survive into adult life. Cleft palate can be repaired successfully and the prognosis for normal speech is good.

Differential Diagnosis: There are many forms of genetic disorders that have short stature and disproportionately short limbs. Several are allelic to diastrophic dysplasia, including several forms of atelosteogenesis and achondrogenesis. The craniofacial manifestations of **achondroplasia** are very different from diastrophic dysplasia, as are the radiographic findings of the skeleton.

Distal Arthrogryposis

Also Known As: Arthrogryposis multiplex congenita, distal, type 1

Arthrogryposis is a symptomatic description for multiple congenital joint contractures. Arthrogryposis as a clinical finding is of heterogenous etiology, but there are a number of direct genetic causes for arthrogryposis as part of a syndrome complex. Distal arthrogryposis, type 1 is probably under-reported and is a common cause of talipes equiovarus (club foot). Some cases also present with Robin sequence.

Major System(s) Affected: Musculoskeletal; limbs; craniofacial.

Etiology: Autosomal dominant inheritance. The gene has been mapped in some cases to 9p21-q21, the pericentric portion of chromosome 9.

Speech Disorders: Articulation may be impaired by micrognathia and limitation of mandibular movement. Compensatory articulation patterns often occur because of the combined effects of cleft palate, velopharyngeal insufficiency, limited jaw movement, and malocclusion.

Feeding Disorders: Early feeding is often impaired by airway obstruction, especially in those cases that have associated Robin sequence. Limited oral opening may also make early feeding more difficult.

Hearing Disorders: Hearing is usually normal.

Voice Disorders: Voice is usually normal.

Resonance Disorders: Both nasal and oral resonance may be impaired. Nasal resonance occurs secondary to cleft palate and velopharyngeal insufficiency, combined with limited oral opening which may help to direct resonance out of the nose. Oropharyngeal resonance may be impaired by limited oral opening and micrognathia resulting in a muffled oral resonance.

Language Disorders: Language development is typically normal, as is cognition.

Other Clinical Features:

Musculoskeletal: talipes equinovarus; ulnar deviation of the fingers; clenched hands; digit contractions; multiple joint contractions;

Craniofacial: micrognathia; occasional trismus; Robin sequence.

Natural History: The contractures are present at birth and are occasionally confused for abnormal fetal positioning. The contractures typically respond well to physical therapy and joint manipulation. Cognition is normal, and once the contractures are treated, motor development may be fairly normal, as well.

Treatment Prognosis: Excellent.

Differential Diagnosis: Club foot in association with micrognathia and Robin sequence is seen in Stickler syndrome, velo-cardiofacial syndrome, and Freeman-Sheldon syndrome. Only Freeman-Sheldon syndrome has multiple joint contractures. Joint abnormalities (pterygia) and Robin sequence is also found in popliteal pterygium syndrome, but the joint abnormalities are structural webs rather than musculoskeletal contractions.

NOTE: Distal arthrogryposis appears in this PocketGuide in two forms: Type 1 (this entry) and Type 2B (Freeman-Sheldon syndrome). There are two additional forms of distal arthrogryposis (also known as arthrogryposis multiplex congenita, distal) differentiated in part by their phenotypes, and also by their mode of inheritance. There is an X-linked form (designated arthrogryposis multiplex congenita, distal, X-linked and also known as spinal muscular atrophy) that is almost always lethal. It differs from the other forms of distal arthrogryposis in that there are signs of neuromuscular disease, including loss of cells in the anterior horns in the brain. Distal arthrogryposis, type II (or arthrogryposis multiplex congenita, distal, Type 2) is an autosomal dominant disorder with webbing of the neck, spinal fusion, short stature, and hip dislocation. Both of these forms are rare.

Down Syndrome

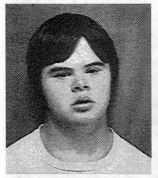

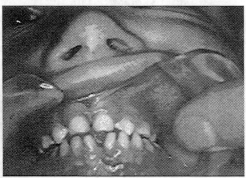

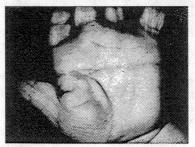

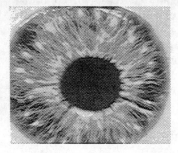

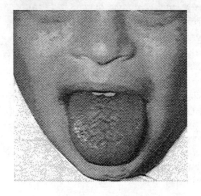

Characteristic manifestations of Down syndrome, including Brushfield spots of the iris (middle right), transverse palmar crease (middle left), small teeth (upper right), and large grooved tongue (lower left).

152

Also Known As: Trisomy 21

Down syndrome is probably the most frequently occurring multiple anomaly disorder in humans with a population prevalence of approximately 1:1,000 people, although estimates vary somewhat. The syndrome was probably first described by Séguin in 1846, 20 years before John Langdon Down developed his theory of ethnic traits and their effect on intellect. Down coined the term "mongoloid idiot," clearly showing his racial biases in his 1866 treatise. As a result, his name has become eponymous with the syndrome. The presence of an extra chromosome as the cause of Down syndrome was not discovered until 1959. Although 95% of individuals with Down syndrome have a complete trisomy of chromosome 21, it is now understood that only a small segment of chromosome 21 at 21q22.3 is responsible for the majority of the phenotype.

Major System(s) Affected: Central nervous system; craniofacial; growth; cardiac; gastrointestinal; limbs; ocular; hematologic.

Etiology: In 95% of cases, karyotype reveals an extra complete chromosome 21. In the balance of cases, the phenotype is caused by

an unbalanced translocation or mosaicism. Individuals with Down syndrome are sterile.

Speech Disorders: Speech is characterized by multiple obligatory distortions secondary to a combination of structural anomalies, including macroglossia, maxillary hypoplasia, malocclusion, and dental anomalies. However, there is an overriding neurological component that causes a slurred speech pattern, but speech rate is typically increased, rather than decreased as one might observe in dysarthria. Speech rhythm disorders are also common and stuttering is more common in Down syndrome than in the general population. There is typically poor phrasing and impaired prosody. Even in cases with minimal structural anomalies or in whom reconstructive surgery has been performed for tongue reduction and malocclusion, the neurologic components persist. Abnormalities of tongue movement are mostly related to motor control problems emanating from the central nervous system rather than from structural abnormalities. Articulation is severely impaired and unintelligible in many, if not most cases. Cleft palate, while not a common anomaly in Down syndrome, does occur with greater frequency than in the general population and may result in compensatory substitutions in addition to the other articulation impairments.

Feeding Disorders: Early feeding is impaired by hypotonia and is often complicated by cardiac anomalies and/or cleft palate.

Hearing Disorders: Conductive, mixed, and sensorineural hearing loss have all been documented in individuals with Down syndrome. It is probable that the majority of hearing loss in individuals with Down syndrome is conductive secondary to chronic middle ear disease. Serous otitis and middle ear effusion are common in Down syndrome because of abnormal craniofacial anatomy, reduced immune function, decreased volume and abnormal angulation of the eustachian tube. Structural anomalies of the ossicles and the cochlea have been reported, including decreased length of the cochlea.

Voice Disorders: Hoarseness is very common and the voice is often of low pitch for somatic size.

Resonance Disorders: Nasal and oral resonance are often disordered in Down syndrome. Hyper-

nasal resonance is common in most cases with cleft palate or cleft lip and palate. Oral resonance is often impaired secondary to tonsillar hypertrophy. Enlarged lymphoid tissue is common in Down syndrome and often leads to upper airway obstruction. Oral resonance is muffled in such cases, yielding a "potato-in-the-mouth" resonance pattern. The neck is often short in Down syndrome, enhancing the muffled resonance pattern.

Language Disorders: Language is essentially always impaired in Down syndrome. Many children with Down syndrome socialize easily and adeptly, often engaging in verbal exchange with children and adults. However, their social skills are typically in excess of their cognitive abilities. As they grow older, it is obvious that language is almost always telegraphic with markedly reduced utterance length and the omission of major components of language. Language skills plateau in childhood and remain stagnant. Auditory memory is typically severely impaired, as is short-term memory.

Other Clinical Features:

   Central nervous system: mental retardation; Alzheimer's disease; hypotonia; cerebellar and cerebral hypoplasia; occasional CNS neoplasias;

Craniofacial: brachycephaly, microcephaly; maxillary hypoplasia; macroglossia; geographic tongue; small ears; overfolded helices; downturned oral commissures; epicanthal folds; upslanting palpebral fissures;

Growth: small stature; obesity;

Cardiac: various congenital heart anomalies, including endocardial cushion defect;

Gastrointestinal: duodenal stenosis or atresia; imperforate anus;

Limbs: brachydactyly; clinodactyly; transverse palmar crease; single flexion crease of the small fingers;

Ocular: Brushfield spots of the iris;

Hematologic: leukemia.

Natural History: Initial presentation is one of severe hypotonia and delayed psychomotor development. With growth and development, social skills develop more rapidly than cognitive skills. Language and speech development are usually severely impaired. There is some progression of psychomotor milestones through early childhood, but there is an eventual plateau with failure to progress. Many affected individuals develop Alzheimer's disease and premature senility. Average life span in Down syndrome is approximately 35 years.

Treatment Prognosis: In individuals with trisomy 21, the prognosis is typically poor for cognitive development. Patients with mosaicism may have borderline or low normal intellect, and some individuals with trisomy 21 may have borderline cognitive function, but the majority are significantly impaired with retardation ranging from mild to severe. However, even in higher functioning cases, there is still some plateau effect. Therefore, it is extremely important to aggressively treat children with Down syndrome early, including early speech and language therapy.

Differential Diagnosis: Down syndrome has a singular and distinctive phenotype.

Dubowitz Syndrome

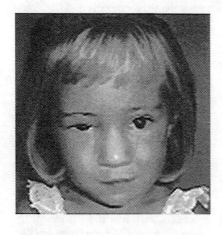

Dubowitz syndrome: Note the right-sided upper eyelid ptosis.

Also Known As:

Dubowitz syndrome is a rare syndrome with multiple speech, voice, and resonance implications that make it a distinctive diagnosis.

Major System(s) Affected:
Central nervous system; growth; craniofacial; gastrointestinal; genitourinary; vascular; endocrine; integument; hematologic; immunologic.

Etiology: Autosomal recessive
inheritance. The gene has not yet been mapped or identified.

Speech Disorders: The onset of
speech is delayed in most cases even though other developmental milestones are typically normal. Articulation may be marked by compensatory articulation patterns secondary to cleft palate and velopharyngeal insufficiency, or by abnormal articulatory placement related to malocclusion. Micrognathia results in a Class II malocclusion and anterior skeletal open-bite secondary to hypotonia and jaw anomalies may also result in lingual protrusion during speech.

Feeding Disorders: Failure-to-
thrive does occur in Dubowitz syndrome secondary to a number of factors including hypotonia, micrognathia and its subsequent con-

tribution to airway obstruction, and cleft palate. Chronic ulcerative mouth infections may also make feeding painful. Frequent vomiting is common, as is chronic diarrhea.

Hearing Disorders: Conductive hearing loss secondary to chronic middle ear effusion is common. Individuals with Dubowitz syndrome have a higher frequency of upper respiratory infections and some immune disorders, thus exacerbating middle ear disease.

Voice Disorders: Voice production in Dubowitz syndrome is high pitched and hoarse. Specific laryngeal anomalies have not been identified.

Resonance Disorders: Hypernasality is common in Dubowitz syndrome. Cleft palate, submucous cleft palate, and even Robin sequence may contribute, but there may also be some neurologic component to velopharyngeal insufficiency.

Language Disorders: Language impairment is variable, but essentially always lags behind motor development. Expressive language is particularly impaired and the onset of speech is essentially always late. There is, however, some eventual "catch-up" and in most cases, language is functional. A small number of patients with Dubowitz syndrome have severe mental retardation and do not develop much, if any, functional language.

Other Clinical Features:

Central nervous system: variable cognitive impairment, ranging from normal intellect to severe mental retardation; hyperactivity; ADD and ADHD;

Growth: low birth weight; small stature;

Craniofacial: primary microcephaly; small face; ptosis; short palpebral fissures; telecanthus; blepharophimosis; high forehead; sparse eyebrows laterally; submucous cleft palate or cleft palate; Robin sequence; micrognathia;

Gastrointestinal: anal anomalies;

Genitourinary: hypospadias; cryptorchidism;

Vascular: aberrant right subclavian artery; internal carotid artery occlusion;

Endocrine: hypoparathyroidism;

Integument: eczema; sparse hair;

Hematologic: neutropenia;

Immunologic: IgA deficiency; IgG deficiency; chronic infections; chronic mouth infections;

Other: increased frequency of malignant neoplasias; somatic chromosomal breakage.

Natural History: Small stature is of prenatal onset. Therefore, although failure-to-thrive is a common feature, the lack of normal feeding in infancy is not responsible for small stature and low weight in childhood and adolescence. Linear growth is always impaired and is a primary feature of the syndrome. Language development is disproportionately impaired compared to other developmental milestones. Many patients fall within the normal range (typically low or borderline) of intellect. The onset of neoplasias occurs in later life and may occur in association with immune deficiency.

Treatment Prognosis: Symptomatic treatment for speech, language, and hearing disorders should be successful if implemented appropriately. Other medical conditions, including neoplasias, have variable outcomes depending on severity.

Differential Diagnosis: Immune deficiency, submucous cleft palate, hypoparathyroidism, speech delay, and hypernasality are all common features of **velo-cardio-facial syndrome,** as is Robin sequence. Skin anomalies with short stature and chromosome breakage is common in **Bloom syndrome.** Short palpebral fissures, low birth weight, and microcephaly are common features of **fetal alcohol syndrome,** but developmental delay is global and often more severe.

Dysautonomia

Also Known As: Familial dysautonomia; Riley-Day syndrome

This neurologically based syndrome is one of a group of genetic disorders that is largely isolated to a single racial or ethnic subgroup. Dysautonomia is almost completely restricted to Ashkenazi Jews from Eastern Europe. This autosomal recessive disorder has a frequency of approximately 1:10,000 among Ashkenazi Jews, but some estimates have the disorder as nearly three times more frequent. This type of frequency for a recessive genetic disorder implies that the recessive gene carriers are common among Ashkenazim, perhaps as common as 1 in 30 people of Eastern European Jewish descent. As the name implies, dysautonomia is marked by dysfunction of the autonomic nervous system and therefore affects all systems, both functional and behavioral, that rely on the autonomic nervous system for input.

Major System(s) Affected: Neurologic; musculoskeletal; gastrointestinal.

Etiology: Autosomal recessive inheritance. The gene has been mapped to 9q31-q33.

Speech Disorders: Prior to the onset of the disorder, speech development is normal. With the onset of noticeable neurologic symptoms, speech eventually becomes slurred and dysarthric. In cases with earlier onset, motor and speech milestones are delayed and speech motor development is abnormal from the start.

Feeding Disorders: Feeding problems, discoordinated swallowing, and possible aspiration are common in infancy and may present as the earliest indication of the syndrome. Aspiration pneumonia may occur repeatedly. Some infants die in the neonatal period from chronic aspiration and airway problems.

Hearing Disorders: Hearing loss is not a clinical feature of dysautonomia.

Voice Disorders: Voice is monotoned.

Resonance Disorders: Hypernasality and unusual oral resonance secondary to dysarthria are the rule.

Language Disorders: Early language development may be normal, but in some cases is impaired in association with global developmental delay.

Other Clinical Features:

Neurologic: hypotonia; hypothermia; positional hypotension; paroxysmal hypertension; syncopy; drooling; lack of corneal sensation; lethargy; absence of overflow tears; breath-holding; absent reflexes; excessive salivation; ataxia; emotional lability; indifference to pain; abnormal perspiration;

Musculoskeletal: scoliosis;

Gastrointestinal: vomiting; irregular bowel movements.

Natural History: Many affected infants initially present as breech births with subsequent feeding problems, including vomiting and aspiration. Some infants succumb in the neonatal period to respiratory disorders. Many of the autonomic nervous system anomalies become progressive and life threatening, with many patients not surviving adolescence and relatively few living into the third decade of life.

Treatment Prognosis: Individual symptoms can be treated successfully in a palliative manner for several years. Speech disorders may respond to therapy until the disorder's progression becomes too severe.

Differential Diagnosis: Dysautonomia is essentially a unique disorder.

Dyskeratosis Congenita

Also Known As: Zinsser-Cole-Engman syndrome

This X-linked disorder involves the progressive growth of skin lesions, particularly on the oral mucosa. It is a progressive disorder with reduced life span because of progressive anemia and the development of malignant neoplasias. Mental deficiency and behavioral anomalies are also a part of the phenotype.

Major System(s) Affected: Skin/integument; growth; central nervous system; auditory; gastrointestinal; skeletal; immunologic; hematologic; ocular; genitals.

Etiology: X-linked recessive inheritance. The gene has been mapped to Xq28. The gene has been labelled DKC1.

Speech Disorders: Initial speech development may be normal, although it is often delayed in cases with cognitive impairment (the majority of patients with dyskeratosis congenita). Once the oral mucosal lesions begin to appear, they may cause significant interference with articulation. Skin atro-phy and scarring often occur, leading to decreased oral sensation. The mucosal lesions may become infected and painful, further complicating speech production.

Feeding Disorders: Neonatal feeding disorders have not been noted or reported. In later life, oral feeding may be complicated by oral lesions, infections, and neoplasias. However, after the onset of the skin lesions, dysphagia may develop because of strictures in the digestive tract related to mucosal lesions or neoplasias. Gastrointestinal hemorrhage occurs from mucosal ulcerations.

Hearing Disorders: Conductive, sensorineural, and mixed hearing loss have all been noted in dyskeratosis congenita. Erosion of the tympanic membrane from the skin lesions occurs in many cases.

Voice Disorders: Hoarseness secondary to laryngeal lesions is common.

Resonance Disorders: Resonance disorders are not common unless oral and pharyngeal lesions or neoplasias are large enough to interfere with pharyngeal or velopharyngeal function. Nasopharyngeal tumors have also been reported that may result in hyponasality.

Language Disorders:
Language impairment is common in the more than 50% of individuals with this syndrome who are cognitively impaired. Mental retardation is a common manifestation of the syndrome.

Other Clinical Features:

Skin/integument: areas of skin hyper/hypopigmentation; skin lesions (plaques) that result in atrophy and scarring; oral mucosa lesions; nail dystrophy;

Growth: small stature;

Central nervous system: cognitive impairment;

Auditory: sensorineural, conductive, or mixed hearing loss;

Gastrointestinal: ulcerative lesions in the intestines, rectum, and esophagus;

Skeletal: femoral head necrosis;

Immunologic: infections;

Hematologic: anemia; thrombocytopenia; pancytopenia;

Ocular: lacrimal duct obstruction;

Genitals: testicular atrophy;

Other: development of oral and anal malignant neoplasias; pancreatic cancer; Hodgkin's lymphoma.

Natural History:
The onset of the growth of skin lesions is typically in childhood, generally by 5 years of age. Early death from neoplasias or anemia occur frequently, often by the third decade of life, although some individuals live into the fifth and sixth decade. The lesions are progressive and the risk for anemia and cancer increases with age.

Treatment Prognosis:
Fair. The disorder is progressive, but individual lesions can be treated successfully.

Differential Diagnosis:
The skin lesions are similar to those seen in Fanconi pancytopenia, Rothmund-Thompson syndrome, and **Bloom syndrome,** but the natural history of this disorder differs from these other entities.

Dysosteosclerosis

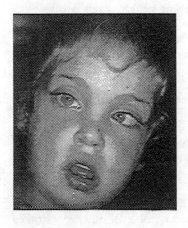

Dysosteosclerosis: Note the strabismus secondary to visual loss, and the flaccid facial appearance secondary to compression of cranial nerves.

Also Known As:

Dysosteosclerosis is a rare syndrome of advancing bone sclerosis that is significant with regard to communication impairment because of the possibility of compression of the cranial nerves. Effects on both speech and hearing have been observed, and in some rare cases, there has been progressive cognitive impairment.

Major System(s) Affected:
Growth; skeletal; craniofacial; neurological; dental.

Etiology: Autosomal recessive inheritance. The gene has not yet been mapped or identified.

Speech Disorders: Speech development is typically normal, but if there is significant cranial nerve compression, facial paresis is a possible manifestation that can affect both articulation and rate of speech.

Feeding Disorders: Early feeding is not problematic.

Hearing Disorders: Progressive otosclerosis is a common finding.

Voice Disorders: Voice disorders have not been reported or observed.

Resonance Disorders: Resonance disorders have not been reported or observed.

163

Language Disorders: Language development is normal in most cases, but may deteriorate in cases with progressive cognitive impairment.

Other Clinical Features:

Growth: short stature;

Skeletal: progressive osteosclerosis; increased frequency of fractures; abnormal growth of the epiphyses, metaphyses, and diaphyses;

Craniofacial: sclerosis of the frontal bone and skull base; hyperostoses of the cranium; late closure of the anterior fontanel;

Neurological: cranial nerve compression; facial paresis; optic nerve compression;

Dental: delayed eruption of permanent dentition; small teeth, deficient enamel.

Natural History: The skeletal anomalies are present at birth, but become progressively worse with age. The onset of cranial nerve compression may begin in early childhood. The onset of otosclerosis is earlier than is typical.

Treatment Prognosis: The osteosclerosis that results in cranial nerve compression can not be resolved with surgery. Therefore, in the most severe cases, the prognosis is poor.

Differential Diagnosis: There are a number of other syndromes with progressive osteosclerosis, including **van Buchem syndrome** and sclerosteosis, neither of which has short stature as a clinical finding. **Robinow syndrome** has short stature as common finding along with mild osteosclerosis, but the facies in Robinow is distinctive and dysmorphic, which is not the case in dysosteosclerosis.

EEC Syndrome

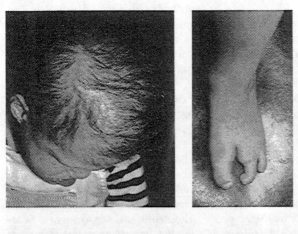

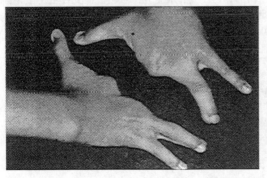

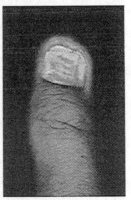

Sparse hair in EEC syndrome (top left) and ectrodactyly of the foot (top right). The hands (bottom row) show ectrodactyly including missing digits (bottom left) and dysplastic nails (bottom right).

Also Known As: Ectrodactyly, ectodermal dysplasia, and clefting

EEC is an easily recognized multiple anomaly disorder because of the combination of clefting, hand and foot anomalies, dental anomalies, and abnormal hair. Because all of these malformations are easy to see by even casual examination, EEC is a syndrome that most clinicians would have little trouble recognizing. EEC is also one of a number of syndromes with mixing of cleft type within a single pedigree. In other words, some individuals in the same family may have cleft palate, while others have cleft lip and palate. The mixing of cleft types within the same family only occurs in syndromic clefting. There is marked variability of expression.

Major System(s) Affected: Craniofacial; limbs; integument; ocular; dental; genitourinary; central nervous system.

Etiology: Autosomal dominant inheritance. The gene has been mapped to 7q11.2-q21.3.

Speech Disorders: Articulation distortions are common in the syndrome because of large gaps caused by congenitally missing teeth and abnormally small and malformed teeth. Maxillary hypoplasia and Class III malocclusion also causes anterior obligatory distortions and lingual protrusion. Cleft palate or cleft lip and palate can also result in compensatory articulation patterns.

Feeding Disorders: Early feeding may be minimally complicated by cleft palate.

Hearing Disorders: Conductive hearing loss secondary to middle ear effusion occurs secondary to cleft palate. Occasional ossicular anomalies and sensorineural hearing loss have been reported, but are not common in the syndrome.

Voice Disorders: Hoarseness is common.

Resonance Disorders: Hypernasality secondary to cleft palate and resultant velopharyngeal insufficiency may occur. Choanal atresia has been reported as an infrequent finding and results in hyponasality.

Language Disorders: Language development is usually normal, but cognitive impairment and language delay occurs as a low frequency anomaly (approximately 5 to 10% of cases). The author has had one patient who did not develop expressive language and was severely retarded.

Other Clinical Features:

Craniofacial: cleft palate plus/minus cleft lip; maxillary hypoplasia; choanal atresia; microcephaly;

Limbs: ectrodactyly; cleft hands and feet; syndactyly; missing digits;

Integument: hypohydrosis; thin skin; very fair skin; very light, brittle hair; sparse hair; hypoplastic or absent nails; sparse eyelashes and eyebrows;

Ocular: sensitivity to light (photophobia); dacryocystitis; absent punctae; inflammation and infection of the eyelids;

Dental: missing teeth; malformed teeth; thin enamel;

Genitourinary: renal anomalies; ureter anomalies; hydronephrosis; hydroureter; cryptorchidism; hypospadias;

Central nervous system: cognitive impairment.

Natural History: The anomalies associated with EEC syndrome are present at birth and nonprogressive. Hoarseness is related to hypohydrosis and lack of lubrication of the vocal cords. Maxillary hypoplasia is always present, but gets relatively more severe as the mandible grows in adolescence. By late teen years, midface deficiency is severe. In part, there is lack of vertical growth of the maxilla because of deficient alveolar bone because of missing and small teeth with small roots.

Treatment Prognosis: In cases without cognitive impairment, the prognosis is good. Speech disorders can be treated as in other patients with clefts. Denitition can be restored with prosthetics or implants. There is no contraindication to maxillary surgery in late teen years.

Differential Diagnosis: Ectodermal dysplasia and clefting occur in **AEC syndrome** and **Rapp-Hodgkin syndrome**. However, neither of these syndromes has digit reduction or clefting of the hands and feet.

Ellis-van Creveld Syndrome

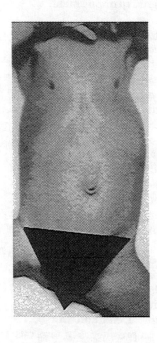

Ellis-van Creveld syndrome: Narrow chest with pectus carinatum in young child.

Also Known As: Chondroecto-dermal dysplasia; mesoectodermal dysplasia

Ellis-van Creveld syndrome is a syndrome of short stature and ec-todermal dysplasia that occurs most often in the Pennsylvania Dutch population (the Amish). The majority of cases have been re-ported from Lancaster County, Pennsylvania, but the syndrome does occur in other ethnic and racial subgroups. Estimated population prevalence is 1:100,000.

Major System(s) Affected: Growth; skeletal; limbs; integu-ment; dentofacial; cardiac; genitals.

Etiology: Autosomal recessive inheritance. The gene has been mapped to 4p16.

Speech Disorders: Articula-tion may be distorted by small or missing teeth, early tooth loss, and a short midline upper labial frenulum.

Feeding Disorders: Feeding has not been reported to be disordered.

Hearing Disorders: Hearing is normal.

Voice Disorders: Voice is normal.

Resonance Disorders: Resonance is normal.

Language Disorders: Mental retardation is an occasional finding in Ellis-van Creveld syndrome, but in mentally normal patients language development is normal.

Other Clinical Features:

Growth: short stature with disproportionately short limbs; average adult height is under 5 feet and may be under 4 feet;

Skeletal: short limbs; osteochondrodysplasia;

Limbs: shortening of the forearms and lower leg; postaxial polydactyly; brachydactyly; tibial hypoplasia; genu valgum;

Integument: hypoplastic nails;

Dentofacial: short midline maxillary frenulum causing a notch in the upper lip (not a cleft) and obliteration of the buccal sulcus in the midline of the upper lip; small teeth, congenitally missing teeth;

Cardiac: atrial septal defect; single atrium;

Genitals: hypospadias.

Natural History: The anomalies obvious at birth and although not progressive, the lack of limb growth results in short stature appearing worse with age.

Treatment Prognosis: The short maxillary frenulum can be surgically treated and dentition can be restored prosthetically or with implants. The prognosis for normal speech is excellent.

Differential Diagnosis: Other chondrodystrophies with similar skeletal findings, such as **achondroplasia** and **cartilage-hair hypoplasia** are distinctly different from Ellis-van Creveld syndrome. In particular, the facial appearance in Ellis-van Creveld syndrome is normal as is head size.

Escobar Syndrome

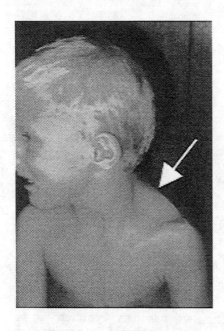

Pterygium coli (arrow) in Escobar syndrome.

Also Known As: Pterygium syndrome; multiple pterygium syndrome; pterygium colli syndrome

There is some confusion in the naming of this syndrome, and probably a number of different multiple anomaly disorders have come under the label of "multiple pterygium syndrome." This author prefers the label of Escobar syndrome in recognition of Victor Escobar's detailed delineation of the syndrome over 2 decades ago. The use of pterygium syndrome, multiple pterygium syndrome, or pterygium colli syndrome can be somewhat confusing in relation to other syndromes, including popliteal pterygium syndrome. Escobar syndrome is a distinct entity with distinct differences from popliteal pterygium syndrome.

Major System(s) Affected: Growth; limbs; craniofacial; mus-

170

culoskeletal; genital; cardiopulmonary; gastrointestinal.

Etiology: Autosomal recessive inheritance. The gene has not been mapped or identified.

Speech Disorders: Articulation is impaired by a combination of factors. There is usually severe micrognathia with limited oral opening and restriction of mandibular range of motion. Cleft palate with or without cleft lip may add compensatory articulation patterns. Most common is severe tongue-backing related to the limited mandibular motion.

Feeding Disorders: Early feeding is often impaired by airway obstruction and glossoptosis.

Hearing Disorders: Conductive hearing loss is common.

Voice Disorders: Voice disorders have not been reported or observed.

Resonance Disorders: Both oral and nasal resonance disorders may occur. Hypernasality occurs secondary to cleft palate. Oral resonance is impaired by retropositioning of the mandible and tongue causing a severely muffled oral resonance and may assist in directing resonance through the nasal cavity because of limited oral opening.

Language Disorders: Language development is normal.

Other Clinical Features:

Growth: small stature;

Limbs: severe contractures of the fingers and toes; multiple joint contractures; rocker-bottom feet; syndactyly;

Craniofacial: micrognathia; cleft palate plus/minus cleft lip; limited oral opening; low posterior hair line; down-slanting palpebral fissures; down-turned oral commissures;

Musculoskeletal: multiple pterygia , including the neck, popliteal spaces, elbows; vertebral fusions; kyphoscoliosis; pectus carinatum; muscle hypoplasia;

Genital: cryptorchidism; small male genitals; absence of the labia majora; small clitoris;

Cardiopulmonary: pulmonary restriction; dilated aortic root; small heart;

Gastrointestinal: short ascending colon; absent appendix.

Natural History: The contractures are present at birth, but become progressively worse with growth. Muscle wasting follows.

Treatment Prognosis: The pterygia can not be surgically removed because vital nerves and vasculature are integrated within them. Oral management is also difficult because of persistent posterior pulling by the pterygia colli.

Differential Diagnosis: Multiple pterygia are also common in **popliteal pterygium syndrome,** but do not occur in the upper body. **Noonan syndrome** and **Turner syndrome** both have pterygia colli, but the heart and endocrine disorders distinguish these syndromes from Escobar syndrome.

Fabry Syndrome

Also Known As: Fabry disease; Anderson-Fabry disease; hereditary dystopic lipidosis

Fabry syndrome has been a recognized clinical entity for over 100 years and is now understood to be a genetic inability to break down glycolipids so that they are stored in some of the body's tissues, specifically the lysosomes of the skin, cornea, and smooth muscle. Dark nodular growths known as angiectases form in the skin, especially on the genitals, knees, umbilical area, buttocks, and mucous membranes.

Major System(s) Affected: Skin; ocular; renal; nervous system; cardiac.

Etiology: X-linked. The gene has been mapped to Xq22. The gene has been cloned and is labelled GLA and is known to be approximately 12 kilobases in length.

Speech Disorders: Storage of glycolipids in the lips and oral mucosa may interfere with articulatory placement.

Feeding Disorders: Early feeding is normal. Feeding later in life may be impaired following cerebrovascular event or strokes leading to dysphagia. Feeding may also be affected by airway obstruction caused by swelling of the upper and lower airway mucosal linings. Chronic diarrhea, nausea, and vomiting are common and may interrupt normal dietary habits.

Hearing Disorders: High-frequency sensorineural loss is common, accompanied by diminished vestibular function.

Voice Disorders: Early voice is normal, but may eventually become hoarse secondary to storage of glycolipids in the laryngeal mucosa.

Resonance Disorders: Resonance may become hyponasal related to growths and swelling of the nasal or nasopharyngeal mucosa.

Language Disorders: Language development is usually normal, but later in life cerebrovascular events may result in aphasia.

F

Other Clinical Features:

Skin: development of angiectases (dark nodular lesions); lesions and swelling of the mucous membranes;

Ocular: surface corneal opacity; vascular lesions of the fundus;

Renal: renal failure;

Nervous system: chronic acroparesthesia; seizures; cerebrovascular events; chronic headaches; dizziness; hemiplegia;

Cardiac: angina; ECG abnormalities; septal hypertrophy.

Natural History: The skin lesions are first noted in late childhood, usually after 10 years of age and then become progressively more numerous. The major debilitating symptom of the syndrome is chronic and intractable burning pain that also begins in childhood and may be brought on by external temperature shifts, exercise, or an illness with fever. These pains also begin in childhood. Renal failure occurs somewhat later and is progressive. Life span is typically shortened to an average of approximately 45 years.

Treatment Prognosis: The disorder is progressive and related to a primary metabolic error. The long term prognosis is poor.

Differential Diagnosis: Syndromes with multiple dark skin lesions include **multiple lentigines syndrome** (LEOPARD syndrome), **basal cell nevus syndrome,** and Peutz-Jeghers syndrome. However, the lesions in these syndromes are qualitatively different than in Fabry syndrome, and are easily distinguished by close examination.

Facio-cardio-renal Syndrome

Also Known As: Eastman-Bixler syndrome

This is a rare syndrome with very few cases described in the literature. There is severe mental retardation and abnormal reflexes indicative of severe central nervous system anomalies.

Major System(s) Affected: Central nervous system; kidneys; cardiac; endocrine; craniofacial.

Etiology: Autosomal recessive inheritance. The gene has not yet been mapped or identified.

Speech Disorders: There is limited or no speech development secondary to severe mental retardation in some cases, and marked delay in more mildly expressed cases. Compensatory articulation impairment secondary to cleft palate may also occur.

Feeding Disorders: Early feeding may be impaired by severe neuromotor delay or cleft palate.

Hearing Disorders: No hearing loss has been identified or reported.

Voice Disorders: No voice disorders have been identified or reported.

Resonance Disorders: Hypernasal resonance is possible in cases with cleft palate.

Language Disorders: There is severely impaired or absent language in many cases. In milder cases, cognition is mildly impaired.

Other Clinical Features:

> **Central nervous system:** hyperactive reflexes; clonus at the ankles; severe mental retardation;
>
> **Kidneys:** horseshoe kidneys;
>
> **Cardiac:** conduction defect; heart enlargement; endocardial fibroelastosis;
>
> **Endocrine:** growth hormone deficiency;
>
> **Craniofacial:** long face; vertical maxillary excess; steep mandibular plane angle; chronic open-mouth posture, cleft palate.

F

Natural History: Developmental impairment is severe and obvious from birth. Chronic respiratory problems persist throughout life.

Treatment Prognosis: In cases with severe cognitive impairment, the prognosis is poor. In milder cases, responsiveness to speech and language therapy is dependent on the degree of cognitive impairment.

Differential Diagnosis: There are many syndromes that feature mental retardation with vertically long face and kidney anomalies, including **velo-cardio-facial syndrome.** Kidney anomalies and mental retardation are also common in **Rubinstein-Taybi syndrome.**

Facioscapulohumeral Muscular Dystrophy

Also Known As: Landouzy-Dejerine muscular dystrophy

Facioscapulohumeral muscular dystrophy is one of the most common forms of myopathy. Only Duschenne muscular dystrophy and myotonic dystrophy are more common.

Major System(s) Affected: Muscular; ocular; auditory; cardiopulmonary; skeletal.

Etiology: Autosomal dominant inheritance. The gene has been mapped to 4q35.

Speech Disorders: Weakness of the facial muscles leads to secondary growth disturbance of the mandible and maxilla with vertical growth pattern, anterior skeletal open-bite, and increased lower face height. Malocclusion is common, and often presents as occlusion posteriorly on the molars with the rest of the bite open. This leads to anterior lingual protrusion and obligatory distortions and substitutions for lingua-dental and lingua-alveolar sounds. Articulation may also be sluggish and slightly dysarthric.

Feeding Disorders: Early feeding is not typically problematic and even with the onset of the muscle disease, swallowing is not impaired. However, chewing may be problematic because of the malocclusion.

Hearing Disorders: Sensorineural hearing loss is common.

Voice Disorders: Voice is typically normal, but mild breathiness may occur.

Resonance Disorders: Hypernasality relative to muscle weakness of the palate and pharynx is common.

Language Disorders: Language development is normal.

Other Clinical Features:

> **Muscular:** facial, trunk, and upper arm muscle weakness;

F

leg weakness may occur later in life;

Ocular: vascular anomalies of the retina; retinal detachment; macular degeneration;

Auditory: sensorineural hearing loss;

Cardiopulmonary: atrial tachycardia; cor pulmonale secondary to respiratory restriction and obstructive apnea; pulmonary restriction;

Skeletal: secondary distortion and deformation of the skeleton, including scapular winging; flattening of the clavicles, and vertical facial growth pattern with steep mandibular plane angle.

Natural History: The obvious manifestations of the disorder may be recognized in childhood, including changes in facial structure, spontaneous onset of hypernasality, general facial weakness, and sensorineural hearing loss. The onset of weakness in the trunk and upper arms may not occur until many years later. Life expectancy may not be affected.

Treatment Prognosis: Hypernasality may be treated surgically or prosthetically, although surgical management must be approached carefully because of anesthesia risks. Dentofacial anomalies may also be treated with orthognathic surgery.

Differential Diagnosis: Facioscapulohumeral muscular dystrophy has similarities in terms of muscle weakness to other muscular dystrophies, but is a more benign form. Hypernasality may be seen in many other neuropathies, including **Steinert syndrome** (myotonic dystrophy), nemaline myopathy, and **oculopharyngeal muscular dystrophy.**

Femoral Hypoplasia Unusual Facies Syndrome

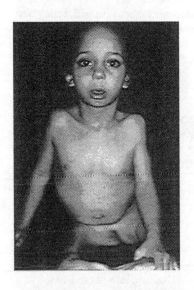 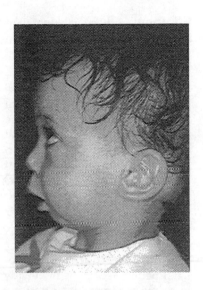

Femoral hypoplasia unusual facies syndrome: Bilateral absence of the femurs and hypoplastic labia majora (left) and micrognathia in femoral dysgenesis syndrome.

Also Known As: Bilateral femoral dysgenesis unusual facies syndrome; femoral-facial syndrome

Bilateral femoral dysgenesis is an unusual clinical finding, but does occur in association with Robin sequence in this syndrome. The syndrome is phenotypically similar to caudal regression syndrome, a disorder caused by the teratogenic effects of maternal diabetes, but is genetic in causation with autosomal dominant inheritance surmised based on several cases of familial occurrences.

Major System(s) Affected: Craniofacial; limbs; genitals; skeletal.

Etiology: Autosomal dominant inheritance. The gene has not been mapped or identified.

Speech Disorders: Articulation is typically impaired by abnormal jaw relationships caused by severe micrognathia and limited oral opening. In addition, cleft palate, often very wide (a U-shaped cleft associated with Robin sequence) leads to velopharyngeal insufficiency and possible compensatory articulation substitutions.

Feeding Disorders: In the neonatal period, feeding is frequently impaired by upper airway obstruction and glossoptosis secondary to Robin sequence and micrognathia. Once airway obstruction is relieved, feeding is typically normal.

Hearing Disorders: Conductive hearing loss caused by middle ear effusion secondary to cleft palate is common.

Voice Disorders: Voice disorders are not a part of this syndrome's phenotype.

Resonance Disorders: Resonance disorders of two types have been observed. Hypernasal resonance secondary to cleft palate and velopharyngeal insufficiency are common. Oral resonance is also disturbed because of micrognathia and glossoptosis with a persistent posterior positioning of the tongue resulting in a muffled oral resonance.

Language Disorders: Language development is typically normal.

Other Clinical Features:

> **Craniofacial:** micrognathia; short lower third of the face; long philtrum; short nose;

> **Limbs:** femoral hypoplasia or aplasia; polydactyly; bifid hallux; low-set thumbs;

> **Genitals:** absent labia majora;

> **Skeletal:** spina bifida occulta; scoliosis; lordosis; minor rib anomalies.

Natural History: The anomalies in femoral hypoplasia unusual facies syndrome are static and nonprogressive. Even with their severe limb malformations, patients may learn to ambulate, usually with assistance (such as crutches). Intellect is normal.

Treatment Prognosis: Excellent. Speech disorders may be resolved therapeutically after correction of physical anomalies (i.e., palate repair).

Differential Diagnosis: Caudal regression syndrome is related to maternal diabetes and presumed vascular anomalies. Patients with caudal regression may have cognitive impairment, a finding not associated with femoral hypoplasia unusual facies.

F

Fetal Alcohol Syndrome

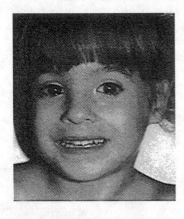

Fetal alcohol syndrome: Note the short palpebral fissures and thin upper lip associated with alcohol teratogenesis.

Also Known As: Fetal alcohol effects; ethyl alcohol embryopathy

Although fetal alcohol syndrome did not become a well delineated diagnostic entity until the 1970s, the recognition of the teratogenic effects of alcohol had probably been understood for hundreds of years. Although clinicians are often taught to recognize the "typical" features of the teratogenic effects of ethanol, the reality is that the phenotype is highly variable because the expression of the disorder is dependent on a number of variables, including:

1. The amount consumed by the mother.

2. The ability of the mother to metabolize the alcohol consumed before it reaches the placenta and developing embryo.

3. The stage of develoment of the embryo/fetus and the susceptibility of the particular tissues developing most vigorously at the time of alcohol consumption. For example, alcohol teratogenesis during the first trimester will result in structural anomalies, but in the last trimester the primary effect will be on the brain which has active development in that trimester, whereas most organ systems and structures have already completed formation.

4. The duration of exposure to alcohol.

Debates about the amount of alcohol that might be "safe" to consume during pregnancy have not typically taken into account these four variables, in part because they cannot be properly assessed in individual cases in a systematic manner. The diagnosis of fetal alcohol syndrome is made based on a history of maternal alcohol consumption (paternal consumption is not teratogenic), so effects are assessed retrospectively in humans and the history provided by alcoholic mothers may not be completely accurate. Although the teratogenic effects of alcohol can be assessed systematically in animals, the effects may not be entirely applicable to human development.

Major System(s) Affected: Central nervous system; growth; cardiac; craniofacial; immune; ocular; genitourinary; integument; musculoskeletal; limbs.

Etiology: Maternal consumption of alcohol during pregnancy.

Speech Disorders: Onset of speech is delayed commensurate with the degree of cognitive impairment. Articulation is often impaired secondary to neurologically based discoordination. Dental spacing problems secondary to small teeth and bimaxillary protrusion with hypertrophic alveolar ridges may cause distortions. Anterior skeletal open-bite may occur secondary to hypotonia. Compensatory articulation patterns secondary to cleft palate and velopharyngeal insufficiency may also be found.

Feeding Disorders: Early failure-to-thrive is common secondary to hypotonia, irritability, airway obstruction, and micrognathia.

Hearing Disorders: Conductive hearing loss secondary to chronic middle ear effusion is common. External and middle ear anomalies may also occur resulting in more severe conductive hearing loss.

Voice Disorders: Hoarseness is common in fetal alcohol syndrome, in part because of vocal abuse in infancy from persistent vigorous crying.

Resonance Disorders: Hypernasal resonance secondary to velopharyngeal insufficiency is common in cases with cleft palate.

Language Disorders: Language impairment is essentially always present. Both receptive and expressive language are equally impaired, but unless cognitive impairment is severe, most individuals with fetal alcohol syndrome develop functional language.

Other Clinical Features:

Central nervous system: mental retardation; learning disabilities (in milder cases); neonatal irritability; gray matter heterotopia;

Growth: low birth weight; small stature;

Cardiac: ventricular and atrial septal defects; tetralogy of Fallot; pulmonic stenosis; dextrocardia; right sided aortic arch; double outlet right ventricle; endocardial cushion defect;

Craniofacial: microcephaly; bimaxillary protrusion; cleft lip; cleft palate; micrognathia; Robin sequence; flat philtrum; short nose; short palpebral fissures; epicanthal folds;

Immune: DiGeorge sequence; immune deficiency;

Ocular: small eyes; small optic disks;

Genitourinary: labial hypoplasia; hypospadias; cryptorchidism; anomalous kidneys;

Integument: hirsutism, especially on the back; hemangiomas;

Musculoskeletal: scoliosis; bifid xiphoid; pectus excavatum or carinatum;

Limbs: hypoplastic nails; characteristic palmar crease; radioulnar fusion; limited joint flexion; polydactyly; small hands and feet.

Natural History: Babies with fetal alcohol syndrome are typically small at birth. Growth then follows a steady, but below normal course. Babies with fetal alcohol syndrome are often irritable and may also be difficult to feed. Developmental milestones are all generally delayed, including speech and language. Chronic upper and lower respiratory infections are common. The infantile irritability does not persist into childhood in most cases.

Treatment Prognosis: The prognosis is dependent on the severity of cognitive impairment and brain malformation. In milder cases, the prognosis is excellent.

Differential Diagnosis: The heart, palatal, immune, and learning disorders in fetal alcohol syndrome are very similar to those found in **velo-cardio-facial syndrome.** Fetal hydantoin syndrome also shares many of the developmental, limb, and cardiac findings.

F

FG Syndrome

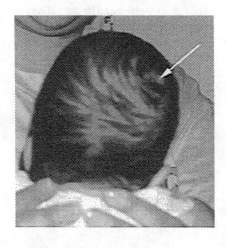

Abnormal head shape with upsweeping hair and abnormal location of the hair whorl in an infant with FG syndrome.

Also Known As: Opitz-Kaveggia syndrome

FG syndrome is an X-linked syndrome of mental retardation with speech, language, and hearing impairment as clinical features. The syndrome is rare, but is probably under-reported.

Major System(s) Affected: Central nervous system; growth; craniofacial; gastrointestinal; limbs; cardiac; integument; ocular; genital.

Etiology: X-linked inheritance. The gene has been mapped to Xq12-q21.31, but not identified.

Speech Disorders: A small number of patients with FG syndrome have severe retardation and do not develop speech, but most are moderately or mildly retarded and develop a characteristic pattern of talkativeness that is probably related to their overall temperament. Patients with FG syndrome are often overly affectionate and friendly much of the time, but then may erupt into temper tantrums and impulsive, disinhibited behavior with occasionally violent outbursts. Their speech may represent a part of their temperament disorder that includes flights of ideas resulting in long strings of emotional speech.

Cleft palate is an uncommon finding in the syndrome, but may cause compensatory articulation patterns when present.

Feeding Disorders: Early feeding is often impaired by hypotonia. Airway obstruction or pulmonary disease may complicate early failure-to-thrive.

Hearing Disorders: Sensorineural hearing loss occurs in approximately a third of cases.

Voice Disorders: Wet hoarseness secondary to lower airway congestion is possible.

Resonance Disorders: Although hypernasality may occur in individuals with clefts, hyponasality is more common. Upper airway obstruction from lymphoid tissue hypertrophy is common and may result in hyponasality. Chronic mouth-open posture and vertical maxillary excess develop from a combination of nasal obstruction and facial hypotonia.

Language Disorders: Language is essentially always delayed commensurate with cognitive impairment.

Other Clinical Features:

Central nervous system: mental retardation; ADD and ADHD; absence or hypoplasia of the corpus callosum; cavum septum pellucidum; hypotonia; occasional seizures;

Growth: small stature in some cases;

Craniofacial: macrocephaly; plagiocephaly; delayed closure of the anterior fonatanel; upsweeping scalp hair; hypertelorism; occasional cleft palate; vertical maxillary excess; protruding ears; overfolded helices;

Gastrointestinal: chronic constipation; imperforate or stenotic anus; megacolon;

Limbs: hypertrophic toe pads; broad thumbs and halluces;

Cardiac: ventriculoseptal defect; conotruncal heart anomalies;

Integument: depigmented and hyperpigmented areas of skin arranged in linear streaks;

Ocular: exotropia; enlarged cornea;

Genitals: hypospadias; cryptorchidism.

Natural History: The anomalies are all static and present at birth. Development is globally slower than normal. Language will often develop in a burst of activity in early childhood.

Treatment Prognosis: Prognosis for communicative impairment is typically good. Behavior disorders, however, tend to get progressively worse with age.

Differential Diagnosis: Many of the anomalies in FG syndrome are similar to those seen in **velo-cardio-facial syndrome,** including the heart anomalies, behavior patterns, constipation, and genital anomalies. However, the pattern of inheritance in FG syndrome is clearly X-linked, unlike the autosomal dominant mode of inheritance in **velo-cardio-facial syndrome.**

Filiform Adhesions and Cleft Lip-Palate

Also Known As: Filiform adhesions of the eyelids and clefting

This is one of the apparently single gene disorders that causes cleft palate with or without cleft lip and relatively few additional anomalies. The syndrome may be underreported because the eyelid anomalies, thin adhesions between the upper and lower eyelid, may spontaneously rupture or be divided at birth and therefore not be noticed by subsequent clinicians. Thus, individuals with this syndrome may be classified as having isolated clefting. However, mixing of cleft type does occur in this syndrome. In other words, within a single pedigree, there may be individuals with cleft palate only, and others who have cleft lip. This mix of cleft type does not occur in nonsyndromic clefting.

Major System(s) Affected: Craniofacial; ocular.

Etiology: Autosomal dominant inheritance. The gene has not been mapped or idenitified.

Speech Disorders: Speech onset is normal, but compensatory articulation patterns may develop secondary to clefting. Obligatory placement errors may also occur in individuals with cleft lip and alveolus, resulting in distortions of anterior sounds.

Feeding Disorders: Early feeding may be initially problematic relative to cleft palate, but serious feeding disorders do not occur.

Hearing Disorders: Conductive hearing loss secondary to middle ear effusion is common.

Voice Disorders: Voice is normal.

Resonance Disorders: Resonance may be hypernasal secondary to cleft palate and the potential for velopharyngeal insufficiency.

Language Disorders: Language development is normal.

F

Other Clinical Features:

Craniofacial: cleft palate plus/minus cleft lip; auricles that are adherent to the temporal region;

Ocular: filiform adhesions connecting the upper and lower eyelids.

Natural History: The developmental pattern in children with this syndrome is no different than normal and no different than that observed in children with nonsyndromic cleft lip and palate.

Treatment Prognosis: The minor eye anomalies can be successfully removed and normal cleft habilitation applied to the cleft palate and cleft lip.

Differential Diagnosis: Filiform adhesions have been reported in **AEC syndrome** (Hay-Wells syndrome). However, AEC syndrome also includes ectodermal dysplasia.

Freeman-Sheldon Syndrome

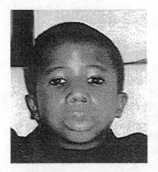
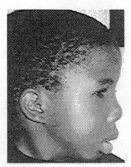
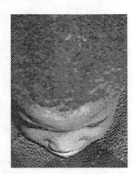

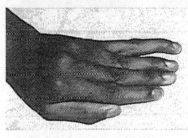

Characteristic facies in Freeman-Sheldon syndrome, including micrognathia and keel-shaped forehead (top row). Note the ulnar deviation of the fingers (bottom).

Also Known As: Whistling face syndrome; craniocarpotarsal dysplasia; Distal arthrogryposis, type 2B; arthrogryposis multiplex congenita, distal, type 2B

Freeman-Sheldon syndrome is one of the genetic distal arthrogryposis syndromes that is associated with Robin sequence and multiple joint contractures with distinctive hand findings. The syndrome is probably under-reported even though the diagnosis is obvious because of characteristic facial appearance.

Major System(s) Affected: Musculoskeletal; craniofacial; growth.

Etiology: Autosomal dominant inheritance. The gene has been mapped to 11p15.5.

Speech Disorders: Articulation is often impaired because of limited oral movement, including restriction of lip, tongue, and jaw movement. Cleft palate is a common finding and may be associated with Robin sequence, resulting in compensatory articulation substitutions. Tongue-backing substitutions are common. A short lingual attachment is also a clinical feature of the syndrome that can cause abnormal tongue mobility.

Feeding Disorders: Early feeding is commonly impaired by upper airway obstruction, Robin sequence, and limited oral opening. Lip and tongue movement are often severely limited resulting in poor sucking ability and failure-to-thrive.

Hearing Disorders: Conductive hearing loss secondary to chronic middle ear effusion is common, especially in cases with clefts and Robin sequence.

Voice Disorders: Voice is typically normal.

Resonance Disorders: Both nasal and oral resonance may be impaired. Hypernasal resonance occurs secondary to cleft palate and velopharyngeal insufficiency, combined with limited oral opening that may help to direct resonance

out of the nose because of increased oral resistance. Oropharyngeal resonance may be impaired by limited oral opening and micrognathia resulting in a muffled oral resonance.

Language Disorders: Language development is typically normal in Freeman-Sheldon syndrome. Cognitive impairment has been reported in a small number of cases, but most patients with Freeman-Sheldon syndrome have normal intellect.

Other Clinical Features:

Musculoskeletal: ulnar deviation of the fingers (so-called "windmill" fingers); talipes equinovarus (club feet); kyphoscoliosis; joint limitation;

Craniofacial: puckered mouth; "keel-shaped" forehead (prominent metopic suture); long philtrum; microstomia; micrognathia; prominent supraorbital ridge; narrow nostrils;

Growth: short stature.

Natural History: The contractures are present at birth and do not get progressively worse with age. Motor development is normal except for the limitations presented by the joint contractures. Early failure-to-thrive is typically related to airway obstruction.

Treatment Prognosis: The contractures do not typically respond completely to physical therapy, but may improve. On occasion, surgery is necessary to improve range of motion. In general, the prognosis is good.

Differential Diagnosis: Club foot and cleft palate with Robin sequence is common in **distal arthrogryposis type 1, Stickler syndrome,** and **velo-cardio-facial syndrome.** Joint abnormalities are also found in **Kniest syndrome.** However, the facial appearance in Freeman-Sheldon is distinctive and different from those in these other disorders.

F

Frontometaphyseal Dysplasia

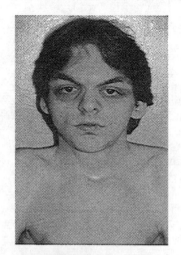
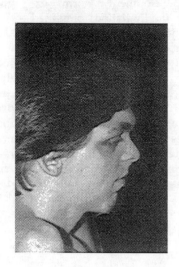

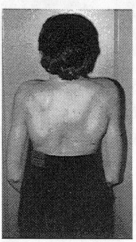

Frontometaphyseal dysplasia: Note prominent supraorbital ridge and kyphoscoliosis (bottom).

Also Known As:

Frontometaphyseal dysplasia is a rare syndrome of craniofacial skeletal overgrowth associated with generalized skeletal dysplasia.

Major System(s) Affected:

Craniofacial; skeletal; dental; respiratory; genitourinary.

Etiology:

X-linked recessive inheritance. The gene has not been mapped or identified.

Speech Disorders:

Speech production is impaired in both articulation and duration. The secondary teeth are typically congenitally missing resulting in over-retained primary teeth and spacing problems that result in anterior distortions. Breath support is weak resulting in weak acoustic production and shortened phrase length.

Feeding Disorders:

Feeding is typically normal in infancy, but with age, airway compromise becomes more severe resulting in difficulties with large, difficult to chew pieces of food. Subsequent dental abnormalities (absence of permanent dentition) may impair the ability to chew certain foods, thus prolonging the amount of time it takes to eat.

Hearing Disorders:

Mixed hearing loss is a consistent finding resulting from the combination of skeletal anomalies and mastoid bone anomalies.

Voice Disorders:

Hoarseness and breathiness are common.

Resonance Disorders:

Resonance may be normal, or occasionally hyponasal secondary to nasal obstruction.

Language Disorders:

Language and cognition are typically normal.

Other Clinical Features:

Craniofacial: prominence of the forehead and supraorbital ridge; short lower third face height with a prominent chin; multiple skeletal hyperostoses; sclerosis of the cranial bones;

Skeletal: metaphyseal dysplasia; kyphoscoliosis; progressive joint limitation and contractions; pectus carinatum;

Dental: congenitally missing permanent dentition; over-retained primary teeth;

Respiratory: pulmonary restriction; tracheal stenosis; subglottic stenosis; obstructive sleep apnea;

Genitourinary: cryptorchidism; hydronephrosis.

Natural History: Pulmonary restriction and subsequent poor breath support are progressive and related to severe deformity of the spine and ribs from progressive skeletal dysplasia. Hearing loss is progressive. Chronic middle ear disease may also occur. Tracheal and subglottic stenoses begin in the second decade of life and become progressively worse. Obstructive sleep apnea also may begin in the second decade of life and is related to both craniofacial anomalies and lower airway anomalies.

Treatment Prognosis: Symptomatic treatment and palliative treatment can be beneficial because the progression of the disorder is not as rapid as in some other bony overgrowth syndromes. Of primary importance is good airway support. Therefore, efforts to limit the kyphoscoliosis should be made.

Differential Diagnosis: Cranio-metaphyseal dysplasia is similar, but the extracranial skeletal findings involve more metaphyseal flaring. In frontometaphyseal dysplasia, the prominence of the supra-orbital ridge is a striking and distinctive feature.

GAPO Syndrome

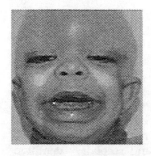

GAPO syndrome: Note alopecia, prominent forehead, and wide mouth.

Also Known As: Growth retardation, Alopecia, Pseudoanaodontia, and Optic atrophy

This autosomal recessive syndrome has a distinctive phenotype with unusual dental findings. Speech is affected by failure for the teeth to erupt.

Major System(s) Affected: Growth; craniofacial; dental; ocular; integument; skeletal; vascular; genitourinary; immune.

Etiology: Autosomal recessive inheritance. The gene has not been mapped or identified.

Speech Disorders: Articulation is distorted by the combined effects of unerupted teeth, maxillary hypoplasia, and an over-rotated mandible that shortens the height of the lower face. The distortions are obligatory because of absence of dental occlusion.

Feeding Disorders: Feeding may be impaired in infancy by upper airway obstruction related to choanal stenosis. In later life, diet may be restricted because of a lack of dental eruption unless appropriate dental therapy or prostheses are applied.

Hearing Disorders: Hearing is normal.

Voice Disorders: Voice is normal.

Resonance Disorders: Resonance is normal.

Language Disorders: Language development is normal.

Other Clinical Features:

Growth: short stature;

Craniofacial: high, prominent forehead; maxillary hypoplasia; short lower third of the face related to mandibular overclosure; choanal stenosis; delayed closure of the anterior fontanel;

Dental: lack of eruption of both the primary and secondary dentition;

Ocular: optic atrophy; glaucoma; keratoconus;

Integument: alopecia;

Skeletal: delayed bone age;

Vascular: veinous drainage anomalies in the brain; prominent scalp veins;

Genitourinary: hypogonadism;

Immune: recurrent infections.

Natural History: Birth weight is normal although length tends to be shorter than normal. Hair is typically present at birth and is lost afterward with most patients having total alopecia in early childhood. Dentition never erupts and both the primary and secondary dentition are retained in both jaws. The anterior fontanel remains patent. Short stature becomes evident in infancy with retarded linear growth.

Treatment Prognosis: Dental treatment is recommended for tooth replacement.

Differential Diagnosis: Alopecia is a common finding in progeria; **AEC syndrome, Hallerman-Streiff syndrome,** and **Rapp-Hodgkin syndrome.** However, the rest of the phenotypes in these other syndromes differ significantly from GAPO syndrome.

Golabi-Rosen Syndrome

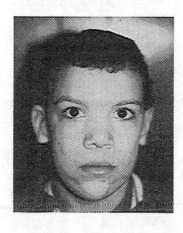

Golabi-Rosen syndrome: Note broad forehead secondary to macrocephaly and mild hypertelorism.

Also Known As: Simpson dysmorphia syndrome; Simpson-Golabi-Behmel syndrome; bulldog syndrome

Golabi-Rosen syndrome is a rare overgrowth syndrome with coarse facial appearance and variable cognitive status, ranging from normal intellect to severe retardation.

Major System(s) Affected: Growth; craniofacial; ocular; limbs; central nervous system; musculoskeletal; cardiopulmonary; gastrointestinal; genitourinary; metabolic.

Etiology: X-linked inheritance. The gene has been mapped to Xq26 and has been designated GPC3 for glypican-3, a gene that controls growth in embryonic mesoderm. The gene acts in synergy with IGF2 (insulin growth factor 2) that is a factor in the expression of **Beckwith-Wiedemann syndrome,** another overgrowth disorder.

Speech Disorders: Articulation is often disordered related to hypotonia and macroglossia.

Feeding Disorders: Early feeding may be problematic related to hypotonia, airway obstruction, pulmonary insufficiency, and some patients have gut anomalies including malrotation.

Hearing Disorders: Hearing is normal.

Voice Disorders: Voice is low pitched and often hoarse. The hoarseness is typically wet.

Resonance Disorders: Hypernasality occurs in cases with cleft palate or submucous cleft palate, or in patients with severe hypotonia.

Language Disorders: Language is typically delayed and impaired. Speech and language do develop in the large majority of patients and the language impairment is usually commensurate with cognitive development.

Other Clinical Features:

Growth: overgrowth and large stature; high birth weight; increased birth length; mild obesity;

Craniofacial: mandibular prognathism; large mouth; macrocephaly; mild hypertelorism; macroglossia; anterior skeletal open-bite; cleft palate (often submucous); occasional cleft lip; notch in midline of lower lip; ankyloglossia;

Ocular: retinal coloboma; cataract; strabismus; retinopathy;

Limbs: broad hands; postaxial polydactyly; syndactyly of index and middle fingers;

Central nervous system: hypotonia; variable cognitive impairment; occasional seizures; clumsy gait;

Musculoskeletal: winged scapulae; short neck; pectus excavatum; supernumerary ribs; advanced bone age;

Cardiopulmonary: pulmonary hypertension; ventriculoseptal defect; pulmonic stenosis;

Gastrointestinal: diaphragmatic hernia; Meckel diverticulum; malrotation of the gut; enlarged spleen;

Genitourinary: large kidneys; cryptorchidism; hypospadias;

Metabolic: neonatal hypoglycemia;

Other: supernumerary nipples; hypoplastic fingernails on the index fingers.

Natural History: Birth weight and length are larger than normal and increased growth continues into adolescence. Hypotonia is more severe in infancy and early childhood and muscle tone improves with age.

Treatment Prognosis: The prognosis for normal speech is good if cognitive impairment is not too severe. Complete habilitation may involve both speech therapy and surgical management of the palate and ankyloglossia. Ortho-dontics or orthognathic surgery may also be necessary.

Differential Diagnosis: Beckwith-Wiedemann syndrome has significant phenotypic overlap with Golabi-Rosen syndrome, as mentioned above. Overgrowth is also common in Sotos syndrome, but the craniofacial findings are different and Sotos syndrome does not have polydactyly as a feature. Prader-Willi syndrome involves obesity and hypotonia, but not linear overgrowth.

Goldberg-Shprintzen Syndrome

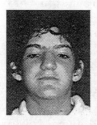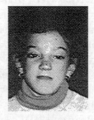

Goldberg-Shprintzen syndrome in an affected brother and sister.

Also Known As: Hirschsprung disease, microcephaly, and iris coloboma

This syndrome of short stature includes submucous cleft palate and digestive tract anomalies. The syndrome is rare, but is probably under-reported because the facial anomalies are not severe.

Major System(s) Affected: Growth; craniofacial; gastrointestinal; central nervous system.

Etiology: Autosomal recessive inheritance. The gene has not been mapped or identified.

Speech Disorders: Speech is marked by articulation impair-ment related to hypotonia, including frontal distortions and lingual protrusion.

Feeding Disorders: Early feeding is complicated by hypotonia and bowel obstruction. The bowel obstruction causes abdominal pain and irritability that can interfere with feeding.

Hearing Disorders: Conductive hearing loss secondary to middle ear effusion is common.

Voice Disorders: Hoarseness and high pitch are common.

Resonance Disorders: Hyper-nasality secondary to cleft palate (submucous) has been observed.

Language Disorders: Language is delayed commensurate with cognitive impairment.

Other Clinical Features:

Growth: short stature;

Craniofacial: upslanting palpebral fissures; submucous cleft palate; microcephaly; brittle scalp hair; midline lower lip mound; large mouth; upper eyelid ptosis; mild orbital hypertelorism;

Gastrointestinal: Hirschsprung aganglionic megacolon;

Central nervous system: mental retardation (usually mild); learning disabilities; hypotonia.

Natural History: Hypotonia and bowel obstruction are present at birth. Developmental delay and speech abnormality become apparent later in toddler years. Short stature is of postnatal onset.

Treatment Prognosis: Surgical correction of bowel anomaly and submucous cleft palate should be successful. Cognitive impairment is static and not usually severe and is therefore amenable to therapy. Prognosis for speech is good.

Differential Diagnosis: The facial appearance is somewhat similar to **Coffin-Siris syndrome,** but the degree of cognitive impairment is not as severe.

G

Goltz Syndrome

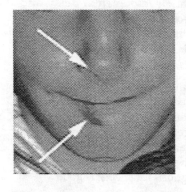

Goltz syndrome: Note mild notching of the nostril (upper arrow) and focal dermal hypoplasia of the circumoral area (lower arrow).

Also Known As: Goltz-Gorlin syndrome; focal dermal hypoplasia

Goltz syndrome is one of the rare disorders that is expressed by X-linked dominant transmission. The syndrome occurs almost exclusively in females, suggesting that the disorder is usually lethal in affected males because they have no matching X chromosome with a normal gene to counteract the mutant gene. The syndrome is distinguished by multiple skin lesions, including focal dermal hypoplasia, the absence or hypoplasia of skin over certain areas of the body at birth.

Major System(s) Affected: Skin/integument; growth; ocular; dentofacial; limbs; gastrointestinal; musculoskeletal; pulmonary; central nervous system.

Etiology: X-linked dominant inheritance. The gene has not been mapped or indentified.

Speech Disorders: Articulation is usually impaired because of multiple structural anomalies, including hypodontia and anodontia. There are fewer erupted teeth than normal, and those that do erupt may have deficient enamel. Spacing abnormalities lead to articulatory distortions, particularly for anteriorly produced sounds. Many individuals with Goltz syndrome develop angiofibromas on the lips and tongue and papillomas of the gingival mucosa. These lesions may be quite large and interfere with articulation or cause discomfort.

Feeding Disorders: Infant feeding is usually normal because the oral angiofibromas usually occur after birth. In childhood, patients form angiofibromas of both the oral cavity and the anus. Feeding and defecating may become painful. Children may avoid bowel movements, giving them abdominal discomfort that may cause them to eat less. Esophageal papillomas may also form, causing discomfort and stricture resulting in vomiting or choking.

Hearing Disorders: Hearing is normal in Goltz syndrome.

Voice Disorders: Hoarseness is a common manifestation of Goltz syndrome.

Resonance Disorders: Resonance is normal.

Language Disorders: Language development is normal in most cases, but impaired in those individuals who express cognitive impairment (less than 20% of cases).

Other Clinical Features:

Skin/integument: focal dermal hypoplasia; angiofibromas and papillomas of the lips, tongue, gingiva, and anus; hyperpigmentation; telangiectasias; subcutaneous deposits of fatty tissue; hypoplastic or absent fingernails;

Growth: short stature, often asymmetric;

Ocular: coloboma of the iris; microphthalmia; strabismus;

Dentofacial: hypodontia or anodontia; hypoplastic enamel; malocclusion; occasional cleft palate or cleft lip and palate;

Limbs: polydactyly; syndactyly; digit contractures; ectrodactyly (split hand);

Musculoskeletal: scoliosis; spina bifida occulta; abnormal bone formation in the long bones;

Gastrointestinal: esophageal papillomas; esophageal stricture;

Pulmonary: laryngeal papillomas;

G

Central nervous system: occasional cognitive impairment, usually mild.

Natural History: Most of the skin lesions (absence of skin, hyperpigmentation) are present at birth, but the papillomas and angiofibromas typically form after birth, usually in early childhood. These growths continue to appear and enlarge throughout life.

Treatment Prognosis: Treatment for the growths is typically palliative removal. In general, the prognosis is good for individuals with normal cognition.

Differential Diagnosis: The syndrome is distinctive, but the skin lesions are similar to those seen in incontinentia pigmenti.

Hajdu-Cheney Syndrome

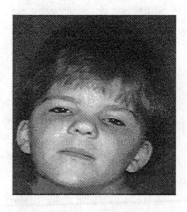

Round, compressed facial appearance with short nose and anteverted nostrils in Hajdu-Cheney syndrome.

Also Known As: Arthrodento-osteodysplasia

Hajdu-Cheney syndrome is a rare disorder that probably represents a connective tissue dysplasia. The primary effects are skeletal and several of the anomalies have a direct impact on speech production. Recognition of the syndrome is critical because of progressive compression at the base of the skull that can cause hydrocephalus and Arnold-Chiari anomaly that may result in death if untreated.

Major System(s) Affected: Skeletal; craniofacial; growth; dental; limbs; central nervous system; ocular.

Etiology: Autosomal dominant inheritance. The gene has not been mapped or identified.

Speech Disorders: Speech is typically impaired by a number of structural anomalies including jaw and dental abnormalities. The dentition is lost early because of alveolar bone resorption and root exposure. The mandible undergoes progressive shortening of the ramus and condyle resulting in shortening of the lower third of the face and micrognathia. Obligatory articulation disorders result from the lack of dentition and severe maxillary overjet. Lingual protrusion is typical. If skull base compression occurs and is not corrected surgically, there may be VIIth nerve compression and facial paresis.

Feeding Disorders: Early feeding is normal. Feeding in adolescence and adult life can be impaired by lack of dentition and shortening of the ramus and condyle of the mandible. The airway may become marginal and result in choking on large or chewy pieces of food. With progression of basilar compression, there may be a loss of sensation in the pharynx and larynx increasing the potential for aspiration.

Hearing Disorders: Both conductive and sensorineural hearing losses have been noted, usually mild to moderate.

Voice Disorders: Low, hoarse voice is a common finding, and breathiness may be present if cranial base compression occurs resulting in vocal cord paresis.

Resonance Disorders: Resonance begins normal, but if skull base compression occurs, hypernasality may result from nerve compression.

Language Disorders: Language development is normal.

Other Clinical Features:

Skeletal: osteoporosis; acroosteolysis; multiple bone fractures; wormian bones; kyphoscoliosis; vertebral anomalies;

Craniofacial: shortening of the mandibular ramus and blunting of the condyles with resorbtion of condylar bone; micrognathia; widely patent cranial sutures; occasional cleft palate; basilar impression causing impulsion of the cerebellum through the foramen magnum; protuberant ears; epicanthal folds; short nose and resulting long philtrum; low anterior hair line;

Growth: short stature;

Dental: loss of dentition and alveolar bone;

Limbs: dislocation of the patellas; joint laxity;

Central nervous system: potential for hydrocephalus; potential for Arnold-Chiari anomaly;

Ocular: myopia; potential for optic atrophy; potential for nystagmus.

Natural History: The anomalies are present at birth, but the skeletal anomalies are progressive. Abnormalities of the skull base begin later in childhood and can become life threatening. Dental loss occurs in adolescence and is progressive as the alveolar bone is resorbed.

Treatment Prognosis: Intellect is normal and with aggressive management, including early detection and surgical management of the basilar compression, the outcome can be good.

Differential Diagnosis: Pycnodysostosis has similar skeletal findings, including bone resorption, fractures and shortening of the ramus, and dental loss. However, the voice in **pycnodysostosis** is high pitched.

H

Hallerman-Streiff Syndrome

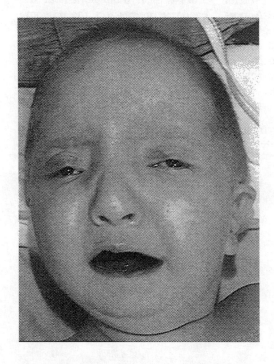

Pinched alar base, narrow face, and missing teeth associated with Hallerman-Streiff syndrome.

Also Known As: François dyscephalic syndrome

Hallerman-Streiff syndrome is a very rare disorder with a striking and singular phenotype that is easily recognized. One of the major problems associated with the syndrome is an extremely small upper airway that often necessitates tracheotomy and often causes severe feeding problems in infancy.

Major System(s) Affected: Craniofacial; ocular; growth; integument; dental; respiratory; skeletal.

Etiology: Probably autosomal recessive inheritance. A gene has not been mapped or identified.

Speech Disorders: Severe micrognathia severely impairs articulation; tongue-backing is a common finding. There is often limited oral opening that results in an inability to maneuver the tongue during speech. The tongue often has a short genioglossal attachment which keeps it positioned inferiorly and posteriorly.

Feeding Disorders: There is often severe failure-to-thrive in infancy related to airway obstruction and micrognathia.

Hearing Disorders: Hearing is typically normal.

Voice Disorders: Voice is usually high pitched.

Resonance Disorders: Resonance is marked by a number of abnormalities, including a cul-de-sac nasal resonance on normally nasal consonants and vowels related to anterior constriction of the nares. Hyponasality has also been observed related to a small nasopharyngeal airway. There is often a muffled oral resonance secondary to severe micrognathia and persistent posterior positioning of the tongue.

Language Disorders: Language and intellectual development are normal in most cases, but a small percentage of cases have been noted to have language delay and mild mental retardation.

Other Clinical Features:

Craniofacial: small face; long, thin nose with a tapered and pointed tip; micrognathia; hypoplastic malar bones; delayed closure of cranial sutures; nasal septal deviation;

Ocular: microphthalmia; congenital cataracts; nystagmus; strabismus; blue sclera; glaucoma;

Growth: small stature;

Integument: selective alopecia along cranial suture lines and frontal area; sparse eyebrows and eyelashes; skin atrophy on scalp;

Dental: hypodontia; malformed teeth; enamel hypoplasia; natal teeth;

Respiratory: upper airway obstruction; extremely narrow upper airway; obstructive apnea;

Skeletal: small ribs; hypoplastic clavicles.

Natural History: All anomalies are present at birth, and the severe micrognathia and small upper airway often lead to severe upper airway obstruction. Failure to thrive is common and tracheotomy may be necessary to alleviate airway obstruction and allow oral feeding. Airway obstruction may result in secondary cor pulmonale, right-sided heart enlargement, and changes in the chest including pectus excavatum. Visual impairment is also evident in the neonatal period. Intellectual impairment is not common in the syndrome, although it has been reported. It is unclear if cases of cognitive deficit are related to hypoxia, or if they represent primary defects in the syndrome.

Treatment Prognosis: The facial appearance is so severely abnormal in many cases that reconstructive surgery is unlikely to yield satisfactory results. It is not known if procedures such as mandibular distraction are applicable to individuals with Hallerman-Streiff syndrome. Speech disorders are directly related to structural anomalies, so that therapy alone is unlikely to remediate the distortions and substitutions.

Differential Diagnosis: The facial appearance resembles that seen in progeria, but is not accompanied by premature senility. Microphthalmia is a key finding in Hallerman-Streiff syndrome, but not in progeria.

Hecht Syndrome

Also Known As: Trismus-pseudocamptodactyly syndrome

This is a rare syndrome that involves limited oral opening and subsequently affects both speech and eating.

Major System(s) Affected: Orofacial; limbs.

Etiology: Autosomal dominant inheritance. The gene has not been mapped or identified.

Speech Disorders: There is limited oral opening that may interfere with the production of some sounds, such as lingua-dental sounds.

Feeding Disorders: Feeding is impaired by limited oral opening, but not typically during infancy. Early sucking and nippling are normal, but once the mouth needs to be opened for larger pieces of food, chewing becomes difficult and modification of the diet in toddler and childhood years becomes necessary.

Hearing Disorders: Hearing is normal.

Voice Disorders: Voice is normal.

Resonance Disorders: Oral resonance may be slightly muffled because of limited oral opening.

Language Disorders: Language development is normal.

Other Clinical Features:

> **Orofacial:** trismus with limited oral opening; enlarged coronoid process of the mandible; short tendons in the fingers resulting in contractions and flexion anomalies; short leg muscles; overly flexed foot; camptodactyly.

Natural History: The flexion anomalies are present at birth and may present as a clenched fist in the newborn.

Treatment Prognosis: Surgical treatment is possible, but there is not a large experience with this problem and a specific prognosis is not known.

213

Differential Diagnosis: Congenital trismus is a rare finding, but limited oral opening is seen in syndromes with microstomia or other contracture problems, such as Schwartz-Jampel syndrome and **Freeman-Sheldon syndrome.**

Hemihypertrophy

Also Known As: Hemihyperplasia

Hemihypertrophy is seen with some frequency in craniofacial centers and maxillofacial clinics because of the facial asymmetry associated with the disorder. Although the population frequency of the disorder is not known, it probably has a frequency of more than 1 per 20,000 people.

Major System(s) Affected: Craniofacial; growth; neurologic; musculoskeletal; genitalia; integument.

Etiology: Unknown. Autosomal recessive inheritance has been hypothesized.

Speech Disorders: Articulation is often impaired by malocclusion. The typical occlusal abnormality is a lateral open-bite that results in some acoustic distortion of lingua-alveolar and lingua-dental sounds. Some patients have central nervous system anomalies that may exacerbate the articulation impairment or cause delayed onset of speech.

Feeding Disorders: Feeding disorders are not common.

Hearing Disorders: Hearing is typically normal.

Voice Disorders: Voice is typically normal.

Resonance Disorders: Resonance is typically normal.

Language Disorders: Language is often delayed because a percentage of individuals with hemihypertrophy have cognitive deficiency. Language delay is commensurate with the degree of cognitive impairment.

Other Clinical Features:

Craniofacial: asymmetric growth of the maxilla and mandible; unilateral vertical maxillary excess; enlarged teeth on the affected side; premature dental eruption on the affected side; unilateral hyperplasia of the tongue and lingual papillae; macrencephaly;

215

Growth: somatic asymmetry; limb asymmetry;

Neurologic: seizures; cognitive impairment;

Musculoskeletal: scoliosis; myelomeningocele;

Genitalia: macropenis; clitoromegaly; hypospadias; cryptorchidism; unilateral enlargement of the testis;

Integument: multiple nevi; telangiectasia; coarse, rough skin on the affected side; hirsutism;

Other: unilateral kidney enlargement; cystic kidneys; nodular hyperplasia of the liver; increased risk of neoplasias including Wilms tumor, adrenal cortical carcinoma, and hepatoblastoma among others.

Natural History: Although mild hemihypertrophy is apparent at birth in many cases, asymmetry becomes more noticeable with age and growth. The affected side becomes progressively larger than the normal side. There may be increased vascularity on the affected side.

Treatment Prognosis: The prognosis is generally good, but it is difficult to predict when the overgrowth will subside unless there is good longitudinal tracking of the patient's growth and bone age. There should be frequent checks for the development of neoplasias.

Differential Diagnosis: Unilateral hyperplasia is seen in **Sturge-Weber syndrome.** The maxillary and facial asymmetry is similar. Some patients with hemihypertrophy also have pigmentary changes of the skin that can resemble **Sturge-Weber. Beckwith-Wiedemann syndrome** also has similar overgrowth characteristics and predilection for Wilms tumor.

Herrmann Syndrome

Also Known As: Photomyoclonus, diabetes mellitus, deafness, nephropathy, and cerebral dysfunction

Herrman syndrome is a rare disorder of hearing loss, neurologic disorders that contribute to speech and language impairment, and endocrine disease. The hearing loss is apparently caused by cochlear degeneration. This condition should not be confused with another disorder labeled as Herrmann syndrome that involves craniofacial and limb anomalies.

Major System(s) Affected: Endocrine; auditory; central nervous system; renal.

Etiology: The syndrome has been described as an autosomal dominant disorder because of vertical transmission on pedigree analysis. However, all cases have been inherited maternally and the symptoms are similar in some respects to other mitochondrial disorders. This may therefore represent a mitochondrial disorder. The pattern of inheritance could also be consistent with an X-linked dominant disorder, but there is no lethality in males.

Speech Disorders: Speech is dysarthric, sluggish, and articulation slurred.

Feeding Disorders: Feeding is not impaired.

Hearing Disorders: Progressive sensorineural hearing loss of variable severity has been linked to progressive cochlear degeneration. Onset of hearing loss may not be detected until the third or fourth decade of life.

Voice Disorders: Voice is normal.

Resonance Disorders: Resonance is mixed hyper-hyponasal of the type often seen in individuals with dysarthria.

Language Disorders: The onset of language is typically normal, but with age, there may be deterioration of function in association with seizures, dementia, and ataxia.

Other Clinical Features:

Endocrine: diabetes mellitus;

Auditory: progressive sensorineural hearing loss;

Central nervous system: photomyoclonic seizures; focal motor seizures; ataxia; nystagmus; dementia; depression;

Renal: nephropathy.

Natural History: The development and progression of Herrmann syndrome is highly variable. In some cases, the onset is very late and the progression slow so that the overall effect is mild. In other cases, the onset is earlier and the progression more rapid with the disorder resulting in early demise.

Treatment Prognosis: In milder cases, palliative treatment is sufficient. In more severe cases, the progression of the disorder is inevitable and treatment is likely to have short-term benefit.

Differential Diagnosis: Refsum syndrome has the association of progressive neurologic impairment and sensorineural deafness, but also has progressive skin anomalies and visual impairment. There are other mitochondrial disorders with similar presentations, including MERRF syndrome (Mitochondrial encephalopathy, myoclonus Epilepsy, Ragged-Red Fibers, and sensorineural hearing loss.

HMC Syndrome

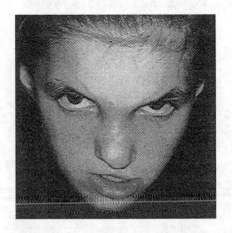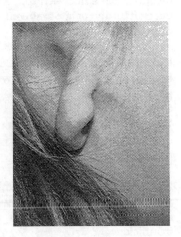

Note cleft and facial asymmetry associated with HMC syndrome (left) with microtia (right).

Also Known As: Hypertelorism, Microtia, Clefting syndrome; Bixler syndrome

HMC syndrome is a rare, but probably under-reported syndrome that features craniofacial anomalies, conductive hearing loss, and renal anomalies. The syndrome may not be diagnosed frequently because many of its features overlap other easily recognized syndromes that are commonly seen in busy craniofacial centers.

Major System(s) Affected: Craniofacial; renal; musculoskeletal; cardiac; central nervous system.

Etiology: Autosomal recessive inheritance. The gene has not been mapped or identified.

Speech Disorders: Speech onset may be delayed. Malocclusion occurs in essentially all cases including lateral open-bite resulting in obligatory distortions or substitutions.

H

Feeding Disorders: Feeding disorders have not been reported, but cleft lip and palate may complicate early feeding attempts.

Hearing Disorders: Conductive hearing loss, maximal in ears with grade III microtia.

Voice Disorders: Voice has not been reported or observed to be abnormal.

Resonance Disorders: Resonance is hypernasal in cases with clefts that develop velopharyngeal insufficiency.

Language Disorders: Language impairment is commensurate with the degree of cognitive impairment.

Other Clinical Features:

> **Craniofacial:** hypertelorism; microtia; cleft lip and palate; facial asymmetry; micrognathia; microstomia; broad or bifid nasal tip; microcephaly;
>
> **Renal:** ectopic kidney; ureter stenosis;
>
> **Musculoskeletal:** vertebral anomalies; hypoplasia of the thenar muscle;

Cardiac: ASD;

Central nervous system: cognitive impairment.

Natural History: The anomalies are present at birth. Facial asymmetry may become more pronounced with age because the more severely affected side of the face will grow more slowly than the normal side.

Treatment Prognosis: Surgical management can resolve the craniofacial anomalies and, together with speech therapy, can result in resolution of speech impairment. Language correction is in large part dependent on the degree of cognitive impairment.

Differential Diagnosis: HMC syndrome has phenotypic overlap with two other syndromes often seen in craniofacial centers, including **oculo-auriculo-vertebral spectrum** (facial asymmetry, microtia, and clefting), and **craniofrontonasal dysplasia syndrome** (hypertelorism, broad/bifid nose, cleft lip/palate).

Holoprosencephaly

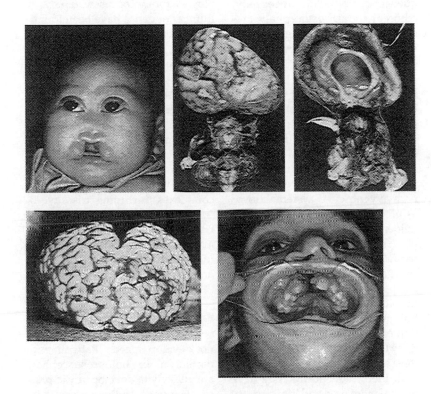

Facial expression of premaxillary agenesis type of holoprosencephaly and the associated brain anomalies (top row). At center is the brain of this baby who expired at 5 weeks of age. Note the lack of hemispheric differentiation and the presence of a single large central ventricle (right). The brain at the bottom left is an example of partially lobar holoprosencephaly with partial hemispheric differentiation. At bottom right is a milder expression with a single central incisor and near midline cleft of the primary palate.

Also Known As: DeMyer sequence; cyclopia; ethmocephaly; cebocephaly; arrhinencephaly; premaxillary agenesis; single central incisor syndrome; Kallmann syndrome

Holoprosencephaly is a term used to describe a spectrum of disorders that involve primary brain anomalies of varying severity. In the most severe cases, there is a complete lack of septation of the brain resulting in a single holosphere without a normal ventricular system, known as alobar holoprosencephaly. In milder cases, there may be complete septation of the brain with partial absence or hypoplasia of some of the communicating tracts, and perhaps lack of development of the olfactory bulbs, known as lobar holoprosencephaly. Partial septation of the brain is known as partially lobar holoprosencephaly. The most severe forms are incompatible with life. Milder forms may have normal mentation and life span, but may exhibit growth deficiency (related to pituitary hypoplasia) or absence of the sense of smell.

Major System(s) Affected: Craniofacial; central nervous system; genitals; growth; endocrine; ocular.

Etiology: There are multiple etiologies for holoprosencephaly. A number of genes have been identified that result in this disorder, including deletions at 2p21, 7q36, 18p11, and 21q22.3. A number of single gene syndromes give rise to holoprosencephaly as a secondary sequence, including Meckel syndrome, **velo-cardio-facial syndrome,** and **Kallmann syndrome** among others. Chromosomal disorders may also result in holoprosencephaly as part of their symptom complexes, including trisomy 13, trisomy 18, and triploidy. Interstitial and terminal deletions have also resulted in holoprosencephaly, including deletions of 18p, 13q, and 2p.

Speech Disorders: Patients with lobar holoprosencephaly do not develop speech. Patients with partially alobar holoprosencephaly are unlikely to develop any expressive language. Individuals with lobar holoprosencephaly may develop speech, and may even have normal intellect. In individuals who do develop speech, many are likely to have malocclusions, maxillary hypoplasia, class III malocclusions, and missing teeth leading to obligatory articulation errors.

Feeding Disorders: Feeding is severely impaired in cases with more severe brain anomalies. Failure-to-thrive is the rule based on severe neurologic abnormalities, including hypertonicity and spasticity with severe irritability.

Hearing Disorders: Hearing is likely to be impaired on a central basis in more severe cases, but measurement of hearing is difficult to assess reliably either behaviorally or electrophysiologically because of the severe brain anomalies.

Voice Disorders: Voice is normal in cases with verbal communication.

Resonance Disorders: Resonance may be hypernasal secondary to cleft palate (including submucous) or cleft lip and palate, both of which are common in the holoprosencephalic spectrum. Hyponasality may also occur related to a smaller than normal nasal cavity in some cases.

Language Disorders: Language development is absent in cases with severe brain anomalies. In less severe anomalies, language may still be absent, but is certainly severely impaired. In milder cases of lobar holoprosencephaly, language development may, on occasion, be normal.

Other Clinical Features:

Craniofacial: severe hypotelorism; cyclopia; single nostrils; absent midline facial structures; absent premaxilla with true median cleft lip; abnormal proboscis in place of nose; microcephaly; upslanting palpebral fissures;

Central nervous system: total or incomplete septation of the brain; absent olfactory tracts; absent corpus callosum and other communicating tracts; pituitary deficiency; lack of ability to maintain stasis; seizures; hypertonicity; hyperreflexia;

Genitals: hypogonadism;

Growth: short stature;

Endocrine: growth hormone deficiency; diabetes insipidus;

Ocular: iris, retinal, and optic nerve colobomas;

Other: many other somatic or craniofacial anomalies

may be associated with holoprosencephaly because of the many potential causes and associated malformations with other syndromes.

Natural History: When the brain anomalies are severe, as in alobar holoprosencephaly, the prognosis for survival past the neonatal period is poor. Babies develop central apnea, have difficulty with temperature regulation, and usually expire within days or weeks. Cases that survive the neonatal period may live into adult years but be severely retarded and be in a perpetual cachectic and spastic state. In milder cases, there may be global develop-

mental delay, often severe. Some individuals have normal intellect and their prognosis is excellent.

Treatment Prognosis: Ranges from extremely poor to excellent, depending on the severity of the brain anomaly.

Differential Diagnosis: Binder syndrome has the appearance of hypotelorism and severe midface deficiency that resemble some forms of holoprosencephaly. Midline pseudocleft of the lip is seen in otopalatodigital syndrome. However, holoprosencephaly has distinctive brain characteristics that can be detected with brain ultrasound, MR scan, or CT scan.

Homocystinuria

Also Known As: Cystathionine beta-synthase deficiency

Homocystinuria is a metabolic disorder caused by a lack of a specific enzyme, cystathionine beta-synthase. Cystathionine beta-synthase metabolizes methionine, and failure of this step in metabolism results in mental retardation and other anomalies. The population prevalence of homocystinuria is probably under-reported, but is probably close to 1 in 50,000 people, even though some reports have placed it as high as 1 in 200,000. The expression of the metabolic defect is highly variable, ranging from severe mental retardation to normal intellect. The majority of cases display mild to moderate cognitive impairment in adult life.

Major System(s) Affected: Central nervous system; ocular; musculoskeletal; vascular; integument.

Etiology: Autosomal recessive inheritance. The gene has been mapped to 21q22.3.

Speech Disorders: The onset of speech is usually normal. The onset of symptoms varies from childhood to adult years. In more severe cases, speech may become rapid and disorganized. Mental disorders are common, including schizophrenia, and speech may therefore be forced and rapid. Spasticity becomes evident with progression of the disorder and speech may become dyarthric and labored.

Feeding Disorders: Failure to thrive is common, but may not be evident in the neonatal period. Feeding and swallowing difficulties are most common in the most severe cases.

Hearing Disorders: Hearing is typically normal.

Voice Disorders: Voice may be hoarse or breathy secondary to thromboses and emboli causing peripheral motor deficits.

Resonance Disorders: Resonance is typically normal, but with progression of the disorder, dysarthria may result in hypernasality and unusual oral resonance.

Language Disorders: Language development is often normal and subsequent deterioration occurs secondary to both vascular events and the primary metabolic defect. Eventual strokes are possible, resulting in aphasia. As the metabolic disorder progresses, language is commensurate with the degree of cognitive impairment.

Other Clinical Features:

Central nervous system: progressive cognitive impairment; psychiatric disorders;

Ocular: ectopia lentis (lens dislocation);

Musculoskeletal: thin, lanky body (marfanoid habitus); tall stature; osteoporosis; pectus excavatum; joint hyperextension; joint contractures; scoliosis; kyphoscoliosis;

Vascular: cerebrovascular accidents; thrombosis; embolisms;

Integument: malar flush; erythema;

Other: pancreatitis.

Natural History: In the most severe cases, the diagnosis becomes apparent in infancy and the disorder progresses to severe manifestations of the clinical findings, including severe retardation. In some cases, the onset is not evident until later in childhood. The onset of the potentially fatal complications of thromboses and emboli varies between the teen years and the fourth or fifth decades of life.

Treatment Prognosis: Variable, depending on the age of onset. A number of treatments have been suggested, including the use of folic acid and other chemicals to assist more normal metabolism.

Differential Diagnosis: The physical phenotype is suggestive of **Marfan syndrome,** but the progression of neurologic and vascular symptoms (emboli and thromboses) is different from **Marfan syndrome** where the main vascular anomalies are related to aortic dissection.

Hunter Syndrome

Also Known As: Mucopolysaccharidosis type II; iduronate 2-sulfatase deficiency

Hunter syndrome is the only mucopolysaccharidosis syndrome (or lysosomal storage disease) that is X-linked in etiology. A number of different mutations in the same gene have been discovered and there are two subtypes of Hunter syndrome differentiated by severity. These two forms have been designated as MPS IIA (severe form) and MPS IIB (mild form). The features of Hunter syndrome are similar to those of the other mucopolysaccharidosis syndromes, including the postnatal onset of coarsening of the face, swelling of the joints, cognitive deficiency and deterioration, and respiratory difficulties. For a more detailed explanation of lysosomal storage diseases, see the entry for **Hurler syndrome.**

Major System(s) Affected: Growth; central nervous system; craniofacial; ocular; musculoskeletal; cardiopulmonary; integument; gastrointestinal.

Etiology: X-linked recessive inheritance. The gene has been mapped to Xq27.3-q28 and has been labelled IDS (iduronate 2-sulfatase).

Speech Disorders: In severe forms, early onset of speech milestones is normal, but with the onset of the clinical features, there is an initial arrest of development and subsequent degradation. Articulation becomes sluggish because the tongue becomes enlarged and the palate and alveolar ridges thickened, preventing normal tongue placement and movement. There is also neurologic degradation that contributes to dysarthria.

Feeding Disorders: Early feeding is normal. In childhood, children with the severe form begin to develop both respiratory compromise and anatomic alteration of the oral cavity making a normal diet difficult to tolerate. A change to a soft food diet may eventually be necessary and in the end-stage of the severe disorder, oral feeding may become impossible.

Hearing Disorders: As chronic congestion becomes more severe, conductive hearing loss occurs fre-

H

quently with chronic middle ear effusion complicated by thickened secretions and "glue ear."

Voice Disorders: With the progression of the upper and lower airway congestion, there is a chronic wet hoarse voice.

Resonance Disorders: Resonance is initially normal, but may become hyponasal with age and the progression of the disorder.

Language Disorders: Early language development is initially normal for all cases. In the severe form, language development ceases in childhood and eventually deteriorates in adolescent years. In the milder form, language may remain normal into adult life.

Other Clinical Features:

Growth: short stature (more severe in MPS IIA);

Central nervous system: initial normal development followed by cognitive deficiency, mental retardation being ultimately severe in MPS IIA, but intellect is mildly impaired or normal in MPS IIB;

hydrocephalus (in MPS IIA); seizures (MPS IIA); hyperactivity (MPS IIA);

Craniofacial: coarse facies; thick lips; alveolar ridge hypertrophy; thickening of the palate;

Ocular: papilledema; abnormal retinal pigmentation (MPS IIA); retinal degeneration (MPS IIA); corneal opacities (MPS IIB);

Musculoskeletal: short neck (MPS IIA); carpal tunnel syndrome (MPS IIB); kyphosis; progressive joint stiffness; pes cavum;

Cardiopulmonary: congestive heart failure; right-sided heart enlargement; valve disorders (MPS IIA); myocardial thickening (MPS IIA); coronary artery disease (MPS IIA);

Integument: hirsutism; nodules on the shoulders, chest, and arms (MPS IIA);

Gastrointestinal: liver and/or spleen enlargement (MPS IIA); diarrhea (MPS IIA); inguinal and umbilical hernias (MPS IIA).

Natural History: In the more severe form (MPS IIA), the disease becomes noticeable in early childhood and progresses rapidly with the majority of patients failing to survive past the age of 18 years. Cognitive, speech, language, and hearing functions all deteriorate with age. In the milder form (MPS IIB), the onset is later and the progression slower. Patients survive into adult life with only mild cognitive impairments or with normal intellect and language.

Treatment Prognosis: No effective treatments have yet been found for the severe form. Palliative treatment is indicated in milder cases, including treatment of middle ear fluid and respiratory illness.

Differential Diagnosis: The facial appearance and progressive nature of the disorder is similar to other lysosomal storage diseases and metabolic disorders. There are definitive molecular tests that can confirm the diagnosis of Hunter syndrome.

Hurler Syndrome

Also Known As: Mucopolysaccharidosis type I; alpha-L-iduronidase deficiency

The lysosomal storage diseases, or mucopolysaccharidoses, are a group of genetic disorders involving metabolic abnormalities. These disorders are caused by deficiencies of a number of enzymes (lysosomal enzymes) that have the function of breaking down mucopolysaccharides, also known as glycosaminoglycans (GAGs). Mucopolysaccharides, or GAGs, are large, complex sugar molecules that play a role in the formation of the body's connective tissues. In normal individuals, the GAGs are continuously broken down for elimination by the lysosomal enzymes. If they are not broken down because of lysosomal deficiency, the GAGs are stored in the body's tissues. Therefore, these disorders are progressive and in the more severe forms, early death is expected. Hurler syndrome is one of the severe forms of mucopolysaccharidosis with an early and rapid downhill course. The missing enzyme in Hurler syndrome is alpha-L-iduronidase. Hurler syndrome is individually rare, with a birth frequency of approximately 1:100,000, but as a group, the mucopolysaccharidoses occur in at least 1:25,000 births.

Major System(s) Affected: Growth; central nervous system; craniofacial; ocular; musculoskeletal; limbs; cardiopulmonary; integument; gastrointestinal.

Etiology: Autosomal recessive inheritance. The gene has been mapped to 4p16.3 and labeled alpha-L-iduronidase. A number of other lysosomal storage diseases are allelic to Hurler syndrome, meaning that they are caused by different mutations in the same alpha-L-iduronidase gene. Scheie syndrome and Hurler-Scheie syndrome are allelic forms of mucopolysaccharidosis type I.

Speech Disorders: Early developmental stages of vocalization are normal, but the disease progresses rapidly in late infancy/early toddler years. Psychomotor development is often normal in the first half year of life, and then slows dramatically before 1 year of age. Speech milestones cease to progress and little speech develops. Most individuals with Hurler syndrome succumb in childhood, usually before 10 years of age. Limited sound production is hampered by thickened alveolar ridges, a thickened palate, and chronic upper and lower airway obstruction.

Feeding Disorders: Early feeding is typically normal, but with the onset of noticeable symptoms, upper airway obstruction and advancing pulmonary disease result in feeding difficulty. However, patients with Hurler syndrome typically appear "pudgy" and "puffy" because of the intracellular storage of GAGs. They become very inactive and overall caloric intake need not be large to maintain weight. Short stature results in the weight being disproportionately high compared to length. In childhood, the combination of oral cavity distortion and respiratory compromise make a normal diet impossible, and a change to soft diet becomes necessary. In late stages of the disease, alternative feeding procedures often become necessary.

Hearing Disorders: Conductive hearing loss secondary to chronic middle ear fluid is very common.

Voice Disorders: Wet hoarseness and chronic congestion are common beginning at about three to six months of age, and become progressively worse with age.

Resonance Disorders: Hyponasality secondary to chronic nasal obstruction and enlargement of lymphoid tissue is very common.

Language Disorders: Language development reaches a near standstill by 1 to 2 years of age. The cognitive impairment caused by the metabolic disorder continues to progress until early demise within the first decade of life.

Other Clinical Features:

Growth: short stature of postnatal onset;

Central nervous system: progressive cognitive impairment;

Craniofacial: coarse facial features; thick lips; thickened alveolar ridges; thickened palate; macrocephaly; tongue enlargement;

Ocular: corneal opacities;

Musculoskeletal: thickened, stiff joints; kyphosis;

short neck; thoracolumbar gibbus; hip flexion abnormalities;

Limbs: brachydactyly;

Cardiopulmonary: coronary artery disease; valvular stenosis; right-sided heart enlargement; cor pulmonale; obstructive apnea; pulmonary edema;

Integument: hirsutism;

Gastrointestinal/abdominal: constipation; enlarged liver; enlarged spleen; umbilical hernia; inguinal hernias.

Natural History: Onset of the disorder is usually first noticed before 6 months of age with progressive coarsening of the face, a slowing of motor development, stiffness of the joints, irritability, and chronic congestion. After 6 months, development slows dramatically, and by 2 years, becomes stagnant. Later in childhood, there is regression.

Treatment Prognosis: Extremely poor.

Differential Diagnosis: Hurler syndrome is differentiated from other lysosomal storage diseases and metabolic disorders based on laboratory tests specifying the enzyme that is abnormal.

Hypochondroplasia

Also Known As:

Hypochondroplasia is a syndrome of disproportionate short stature that is allelic to **achondroplasia**, but with a different mutation in the FGFR3 gene. Prior to the delineation of the syndrome, it is likely that many patients with this disorder were diagnosed with **achondroplasia**.

Major System(s) Affected:

Growth; skeletal; craniofacial; central nervous system.

Etiology:

Autosomal dominant inheritance. The gene has been mapped to 4p16.3 and has been labeled as FGFR3, or fibroblast growth factor receptor 3.

Speech Disorders:

Speech production is typically normal, but onset is delayed in the approximately 10 to 20% of individuals with the syndrome who have cognitive impairment.

Feeding Disorders:

Feeding disorders are not common in the syndrome, but early feeding may be difficult in the cases with infantile hypotonia who subsequently go on to develop cognitive impairment.

Hearing Disorders:

Hearing is within normal limits.

Voice Disorders:

Voice is typically high pitched.

Resonance Disorders:

Resonance is generally normal although in some cases there is mild hyponasality secondary to a slightly shortened anterior cranial base and smaller than normal nasal capsule. Oral resonance may also be a bit dampened by spinal anomalies.

Language Disorders:

Language development is normal except for those cases with cognitive impairment.

Other Clinical Features:

Growth: disproportionate short stature;

Skeletal: osteochondrodysplasia; short limbs with

brachydactyly; lumbar lordosis; limited extension of the elbows; limited hip joint extension; bowing of the legs;

Craniofacial: frontal bossing; slightly short anterior cranial base;

Central nervous system: occasional mild mental retardation; occasional infantile hypotonia.

Natural History: Birth weight and length may be low, but in some cases is close to normal. Growth deficiency becomes obvious by early childhood. Adult height is typically about 4½ feet. As the child walks more and more weight is placed on the legs, bowing becomes more obvious.

Treatment Prognosis: Excellent. Surgery may be necessary for spinal anomalies. Lengthening of the limbs, particularly the legs, is possible using distraction techniques.

Differential Diagnosis: Achondroplasia has similar findings but the craniofacial anomalies are striking in **achondroplasia,** whereas facial appearance is relatively normal in hypochondroplasia. Spinal anomalies are similar to those in **spondyloepiphyseal dysplasia congenita.**

Hypohidrotic Ectodermal Dysplasia

Also Known As: Ectodermal dysplasia 1, anhidrotic; Christ-Siemens-Touraine syndrome

This form of ectodermal dysplasia was made famous at the end of the 19th century by Charles Darwin who described "the toothless men of Sind." Darwin described a four generation clan of men near Hyderabad who did not perspire, had only a few teeth, and were bald. The description is unmistakably hypohidrotic ectodermal dysplasia because only the men in the family were affected (it is an X-linked recessive disorder), they did not perspire, and they were congenitally missing the specific teeth known to be absent in this syndrome.

Major System(s) Affected: Integument; dental; craniofacial; ocular; growth; central nervous system.

Etiology: X-linked recessive inheritance. The gene has been mapped to Xq12-q13.1 and has been labeled as EDA.

Speech Disorders: In cases with cognitive impairment, speech is delayed. In all cases, congenitally missing teeth causes obligatory articulation distortions and substitutions. In some cases, there is complete absence of primary and secondary teeth. More often, there are a number of malformed teeth, including incisors or canines, and several molars. There is also marked reduction in alveolar bone height causing shortening of both the upper and lower dental arches resulting in articulatory impairment.

Feeding Disorders: There is reduced oral secretion of saliva so that the mouth is perpetually dry. This can cause difficulty in eating certain foods. Therefore, increased drinking of clear fluids is recommended during meals. The absence of teeth may also require a softer diet.

Hearing Disorders: Hearing is typically normal.

Voice Disorders: Voice is typically hoarse related to dry vocal folds and persistent irritation because of a lack of lubrication. In some cases, voice may be breathy. After long periods of phonation, dysphonia is common.

Resonance Disorders: The absence of mucus producing glands causes dry crusting of the nose, and occasionally nasal obstruction causing hyponasality.

Language Disorders: Language is impaired in cases with cognitive impairment.

Other Clinical Features:

> **Integument:** alopecia; if hair is present, it is sparse, fine, and silky; absence of sweat glands; hyperpigmentation around the orbits; mucous membrane atrophy; absence of salivary and mucus producing glands;
>
> **Dental:** hypodontia or anodontia; if teeth are present, they are malformed, usually conical in shape;
>
> **Craniofacial:** frontal bossing; short anterior cranial base with saddle nose deformity;
>
> **Ocular:** absent lacrimal glands; corneal dystrophy;

> **Growth:** short stature;
>
> **Central nervous system:** occasional cognitive deficiency.

Natural History: Ectodermal dysplasia is often difficult to detect in neonates and infants because of the normal absence of teeth and hair in many babies. The fingernails and toenails in hypohidrotic ectodermal dysplasia are normal so they do not contribute to the diagnosis. In addition, neonate and infant skin is often sensitive to external irritants so that the dryness and local inflammatory response of the skin may also be disregarded as normal infantile skin sensitivity. Therefore, one of the earliest manifestations of the syndrome may be unexplained fevers. Without a normal sweating response, babies have a difficult time cooling their bodies when they are warm or when they are active, thus resulting in an elevation of body temperature. After the normal age of dental eruption and hair growth, the diagnosis becomes evident. All disorders associated with the syndrome are nonprogressive.

Treatment Prognosis: The prognosis is good unless there is significant cognitive impairment. Dental disorders that cause speech impairment may not have an adequate solution because the alveolar bone is so underdeveloped, replacement of teeth by dentures or implants may be extremely difficult. If several teeth are present and can be retained, then prosthetic replacement is possible.

Differential Diagnosis: Many ectodermal dysplasias have deficient or absent hair and teeth, but the degree of anhidrosis or hypohidrosis distinguishes this syndrome from others. In addition, syndromes such as **Rapp-Hodgkin ectodermal dysplasia** and **EEC** have anomalies of the nails, as well as cleft lip and/or cleft palate.

Note: There are also two other forms of anhidrotic/hypohidrotic ectodermal dysplasia with different genetic causes. Ectodermal dysplasia 2 is a rare autosomal recessive disorder with a very similar phenotype to the X-linked form. In the recessive form, there are affected females. The affected males are essentially indistinguishable from individuals with the X-linked form. The gene has not been mapped or identified. Ectodermal dysplasia 3 is an autosomal dominant disorder, the gene being mapped to 2q11-q13. The phenotype is not as severe, with milder hair and tooth anomalies, and hypohidrosis rather than anhidrosis.

H

Jackson-Weiss Syndrome

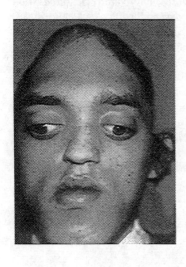

Craniosynostosis, mild hypertelorism, and exorbitism associated with Jackson-Weiss syndrome.

Also Known As:

Jackson-Weiss syndrome is a syndrome of craniosynostosis that is more recently delineated than **Crouzon syndrome,** which it resembles. The syndrome is probably often misdiagnosed as **Crouzon** or **Pfeiffer syndrome.** Its true population prevalence is not known, but it probably occurs with lower frequency than **Crouzon syndrome.** Of interest, Jackson-Weiss is caused by a different mutation in the same gene responsible for **Crouzon syndrome.**

Major System(s) Affected:
Craniofacial; limbs.

Etiology:
Autosomal dominant inheritance. The syndrome is caused by a mutation in the gene FGFR2 (fibroblast growth factor receptor 2) that is located on chromosome 10q26.

Speech Disorders:
Articulation is marked by obligatory anterior distortions related to Class III malocclusion and maxillary hypoplasia. The tongue is often forced to articulate in the mandibular arch

because of constriction and hypoplasia of the maxilla.

Feeding Disorders: Early feeding may be impaired by nasal obstruction and airway compromise.

Hearing Disorders: Conductive hearing loss is an occasional finding.

Voice Disorders: Voice is normal.

Resonance Disorders: Hyponasality is common secondary to nasal obstruction and a small nasopharyngeal cavity.

Language Disorders: Language development is typically normal.

Other Clinical Features:

Craniofacial: craniosynostosis of multiple sutures; maxillary hypoplasia; mild exophthalmos;

Limbs: broad halluces; soft tissue syndactyly of the second and third toes.

Natural History: At birth, some babies with Jackson-Weiss syndrome appear normal. With age, the maxillary hypoplasia becomes apparent and more pronounced as the mandible grows normally. The anterior fonatanel may initially be open at birth even though craniosynostosis is already present in other sutures. The synsotosis is not static, but slowly progressive. Therefore, presence of the anterior fontanel at birth should not be interpreted as meaning that the cranium is normal.

Treatment Prognosis: The prognosis is excellent. Cognitive impairment is not a clinical feature of Jackson-Weiss syndrome. The craniofacial anomalies can be managed surgically.

Differential Diagnosis: Craniosynostosis and maxillary hypoplasia are the key findings in **Crouzon syndrome,** but are more severe and exorbitism is common in **Crouzon** whereas there is only mild bulging of the eyes in Jackson-Weiss syndrome. Soft tissue syndactyly is common in **Saethre-Chotzen syndrome,** but the craniosynostosis and facial anomalies are different than in Jackson-Weiss. Broad halluces are common in **Pfeiffer syndrome,** but broad thumbs are not found in Jackson-Weiss, as they are in **Pfeiffer.**

Johanson-Blizzard Syndrome

Also Known As: Nasal alar hypoplasia, hypothyroidism, pancreatic achylia, and congenital deafness

Johanson-Blizzard syndrome is rare but easily recognized because of the distinctive facial manifestations and endocrine disease. Female cases have predominated, but autosomal recessive inheritance has been confirmed by several pedigrees with unaffected parents and both affected male and female children.

Major System(s) Affected: Craniofacial; growth; central nervous system; endocrine; gastrointestinal; genitourinary; dental.

Etiology: Autosomal recessive inheritance. The gene has not been mapped or identified.

Speech Disorders: Speech production is severely limited in many, if not most cases because of the combined effects of severe or profound sensorineural hearing loss and cognitive impairment. In some cases, there is very limited speech production, especially in the small sample of cases with normal intellect. However, in these cases, "deaf speech" is the norm.

Feeding Disorders: Although feeding is not impaired per se, weight gain is slow because of malabsorption and is often labeled as "failure to thrive." Severe cognitive impairment may also result in hypotonia in infancy. After the age of dental eruption, the teeth are anomalous or absent and chewing certain foods may be very difficult.

Hearing Disorders: Severe or profound sensorineural hearing loss is the rule with Mondini type anomaly of the cochlea.

Voice Disorders: Voice disorders have not been observed or reported.

Resonance Disorders: Resonance is disordered secondary to "deaf speech" in those who have some speech, but in general, there may be a cul-de-sac quality to speech because of a constricted anterior nasal cavity from alar hypoplasia.

Language Disorders: Language is often severely impaired secondary to cognitive deficiency. Many patients have IQ scores below 50.

Other Clinical Features:

Craniofacial: hypoplasia of the nasal alae; beaklike nose; delayed closure of the anterior fontanel; short anterior cranial base; maxillary hypoplasia;

Growth: postnatal growth deficiency;

Central nervous system: cognitive deficiency, often severe; abnormal gyri in the the cerebral cortex; neuronal disorganization;

Endocrine: hypothyroidism; pancreatic insufficiency with malabsorption;

Gastrointestinal: imperforate or anteriorly displaced anus;

Genitourinary: double uterus; bicornate uterus; enlarged clitoris; micropenis; cryptorchidism; rectovaginal fistula;

Dental: absent or anomalous secondary dentition; abnormal primary dentition;

Integument: scalp defects; hypoplastic nipples; coarse and sparse scalp hair.

Natural History: Early failure to thrive is essentially constant because of malabsorption. Coupled with severe cognitive impairment and hypotonia, many infants do not survive, and these effects last into childhood. The pancreatic and endocrine disorders are progressive and become persistent medical problems.

Treatment Prognosis: In many cases, the prognosis is extremely poor, especially those where the cognitive impairment is severe. Even in cases with normal mentation, the endocrine disorders may significantly impair the quality and quantity of life.

Differential Diagnosis: Malabsorption is a feature of a number of syndromes, including Schwachman syndrome, but none have the distinctive facial appearance associated with Johanson-Blizzard syndrome. Hypoplasia of the nasal alae is found in trichorhinophalangeal syndrome and oculodentoosseous syndrome, but these disorders do not have the same endocrine disorders.

Johnson-McMillin Syndrome

Also Known As: Johnson neuroectodermal syndrome; alopecia-anosmia-deafness-hypogonadism syndrome

Johnson-McMillin syndrome is a rare multiple anomaly disorder that has a great deal of phenotypic overlap with other more common syndromes. It is therefore possible that this disorder is under-reported and often diagnosed as another syndrome.

Major System(s) Affected: Craniofacial; central nervous system; growth; genital; cardiac; integument.

Etiology: Autosomal dominant inheritance. The gene has not been mapped or identified.

Speech Disorders: Speech onset is delayed in the cases that show cognitive impairment. Mild micrognathia may occasionally contribute to misarticulations. Cleft palate can result in compensatory articulation secondary to velopharyngeal insufficiency.

Feeding Disorders: Early feeding may be complicated by cleft palate and mild hypotonia in some cases. Otherwise, feeding is typically normal.

Hearing Disorders: Conductive hearing loss secondary to external and middle ear malformations is common.

Voice Disorders: Voice may be hoarse secondary to hypohidrosis.

Resonance Disorders: Resonance may be hypernasal secondary to cleft palate and velopharyngeal insufficiency.

Language Disorders: Cognitive impairment is an occasional finding that contributes to a commensurate delay and disorder of language. Congenital conductive hearing loss caused by middle ear anomalies may also contribute.

Other Clinical Features:

Craniofacial: cleft palate; facial asymmetry; micrognathia; facial nerve paresis;

Central nervous system: anosmia; mild cognitive impairment;

242

Growth: mild short stature;

Genital: hypogonadism secondary to pituitary deficiency;

Cardiac: heart anomalies;

Integument: hypohidrosis; alopecia; café-au-lait spots on the trunk.

Natural History: The anomalies in the syndrome are static and present at birth. Growth deficiency is secondary to the primary hormone deficiency.

Treatment Prognosis: Good to excellent. Patients may be treated symptomatically for all of the disorders expressed in the syndrome with good outcomes, including hormone deficiency.

Differential Diagnosis: The anomalies of the external and middle ear in association with asymmetric facies and facial nerve paresis is found in **oculo-auriculovertebral dysplasia** (OAV), as is cleft palate. However, the integumentary and genital anomalies are not a feature of OAV. Alopecia and hypohydrosis in association with cleft palate is common in **AEC syndrome** and **Rapp-Hodgkin syndrome,** but neither of these disorders are associated with anosmia or growth deficiency with hypogonadism.

Kallmann Syndrome

Also Known As: Hypogonadotropic hypogonadism and anosmia; anosmic hypogonadism; dysplasia olfactogenitalis of de Morsier

Kallmann syndrome refers to a group of disorders with a number of different etiologies that result in the association of anosmia, hypogonadism, and cleft lip and palate. There are a series of allelic variants that are X-linked, and there are probably autosomal recessive and autosomal dominant forms, as well. The X-linked variety is most common with an estimated incidence of 1:10,000 males. The syndrome makes up a significant percentage of males with hypogonadism.

Major System(s) Affected: Central nervous system; endocrine; craniofacial; genital; growth.

Etiology: The majority of cases show X-linked recessive inheritance. The gene has been mapped to Xp22.3.

Speech Disorders: Speech is variable, ranging from normal to severely impaired with neurologi-cal components, including marked dysarthria. In the majority of cases with clefts, there are obligatory misarticulations related to malocclusion, missing teeth, and maxillary hypoplasia. Compensatory articulation may also occur secondary to cleft palate and velopharyngeal insufficiency.

Feeding Disorders: Feeding may be impaired by the cleft anomalies, and there is occasional mild infantile hypotonia. Weight gain may be slow, based on pituitary factors.

Hearing Disorders: Sensorineural, conductive, and mixed hearing loss have all been observed. The majority of cases have been mild bilateral sensorineural losses.

Voice Disorders: Voice is typically high pitched.

Resonance Disorders: Resonance may be hypernasal secondary to clefting and velopharyngeal insufficiency.

Language Disorders: Language may be delayed or impaired

in some cases based on overall mild developmental delay.

Other Clinical Features:

Central nervous system: anosmia; hypothalamic gonadotropic-releasing hormone deficiency; occasional ataxia; occasional cognitive deficiency;

Endocrine: impaired FSH and LH secretion; hypogonadotropic hypogonadism; decreased expression of secondary sexual characteristics;

Craniofacial: cleft lip and/or palate; maxillary deficiency;

Genital: micropenis; cryptorchidism; testicular atrophy;

Growth: occasional mild short stature; gynecomastia.

Natural History: The hypogonadism becomes more noticeable with age, as does maxillary deficiency. All other anomalies are present at birth and static.

Treatment Prognosis: Once identified, the prognosis is good and all anomalies can be treated symptomatically.

Differential Diagnosis: Anosmia and hypogonadism are common in **Johnson-McMillin syndrome,** but **Kallmann syndrome** does not have alopecia as a common finding. Hypogonadism may also occur in milder forms of **holoprosencephaly.**

K

Kartagener Syndrome

Also Known As: Dextrocardia, bronchiectasis, and sinusitis; Siewert syndrome; ciliary dyskinesia; immotile cilia syndrome

Kartegener syndrome is regarded as the triad of situs inversus, ciliary immotility, and bronchiectasis. Situs inversus, the transposition of the body's organs to the side opposite of normal, is a fairly common anomaly that has no practical effect on health. However, ciliary immotility does cause chronic respiratory complications that need careful attention.

Major System(s) Affected: Respiratory; internal organs; reproductive.

Etiology: Autosomal recessive inheritance. The gene has not been mapped or identified.

Speech Disorders: Speech is essentially normal, but can be affected by chronic congestion causing some articulation to be overly "moist."

Feeding Disorders: Early feeding is usually normal unless there is a very early onset of the respiratory symptoms that cause nasal obstruction and respiratory difficulties. In cases of very early onset, feeding may be compromised by respiratory difficulty. In later life, chronic congestion and nasal obstruction by polyps or mucus can cause choking, lack of taste (because of secondary anosmia), and decrease of appetite.

Hearing Disorders: Conductive hearing loss secondary to chronic middle ear effusions and "glue ear"are common throughout life.

Voice Disorders: Wet hoarseness is nearly constant.

Resonance Disorders: Hyponasality secondary to nasal obstruction is common.

Language Disorders: Language development is normal.

Other Clinical Features:

> **Respiratory:** immotile cilia; chronic sinusitis; absent frontal sinuses; bronchiectasis; asthma;

Internal organs: situs inversus; dextrocardia;

Reproductive: male infertility related to immotile sperm.

Natural History: The onset of the respiratory symptoms is variable. Situs inversus is asymptomatic, but is usually detected on normal clinical examination because of abnormal location of heart sounds.

Treatment Prognosis: Typically, the long-term prognosis is very good. With aggressive respiratory therapy (postural drainage, chest physiotherapy, and coughing), longevity is not typically affected. Aggressive use of antibiotics is also recommended for even trivial illnesses. In some severe cases, heart-lung transplant may be recommended.

Differential Diagnosis: Situs inversus occurs as an isolated anomaly with no respiratory disorders. Dextrocardia is associated with a number of malformation syndromes when not accompanied by transposition of the other organs.

K

Kearns-Sayre Syndrome

Also Known As: Oculocraniosomatic syndrome; ophthalmoplegia-plus syndrome; mitochondrial cytopathy; chronic progressive external ophthalmoplegia with myopathy

Kearns-Sayre syndrome is one of a small handful of progressive mitochondrial diseases with neurologic degeneration. The communicative implications are significant in both the speech and hearing realms. Mitochondrial disorders are inherited only from the mother because the genes are located in the mitochondria which are cytoplasmic structures, not nuclear structures. All of the cytoplasm of a fertilized zygote is maternal because the sperm has essentially no cytoplasm, only the nuclear material carrying the paternal chromosome haplotype.

Major System(s) Affected: Growth; ocular; central nervous system; peripheral nervous system; endocrine; cardiac.

Etiology: Mitochondrial genetic alteration, probably a deletion of mitochondrial DNA.

Speech Disorders: Early development of speech is normal. As the neurologic symptoms progress, facial, pharyngeal, and laryngeal weaknesses are expressed. Myopathic weakness is progressive resulting in weak oral contacts and sluggish articulation.

Feeding Disorders: After the onset of myopathy, dysphagia becomes progressive and eventually severe. Feeding becomes progressively more difficult because of poor oral coordination. Eventually, seizures and transient strokelike episodes become frequent and interfere with feeding.

Hearing Disorders: High-frequency sensorineural hearing loss is one of the first signs of the onset of the disorder. The hearing loss is progressive, but the deterioration is slow.

Voice Disorders: Voice becomes initially hoarse, and then eventually becomes progressively breathy and weak.

Resonance Disorders: With the onset of myopathy, hypernasality becomes evident and progressively more severe.

Language Disorders: Language is initially normal. With age and the progression of seizures, there are aphasialike episodes with deterioration of language.

Other Clinical Features:

Growth: short stature;

Ocular: ophthalmoplegia; retinal pigmentary degeneration; ptosis; eventual complete oculomotor paralysis;

Central nervous system: ataxia; hyperactive reflexes; cognitive deficiency; eventual dementia;

Peripheral nervous system: myopathy; peripheral neuropathy; sensory loss;

Endocrine: delayed secondary sexual characteristics; elevated blood sugar;

Cardiac: conduction defects; cardiomyopathy.

Natural History: The age of onset is variable. In general, the earlier the onset, the more severe the progression. The process in unrelenting, although relatively slow. Cardiac conduction defects often result in early death.

Treatment Prognosis: The disorder can not be treated successfully in either a palliative or definitive manner.

Differential Diagnosis: There are a number of mitochondrial syndromes that have associated hearing loss, including Borud syndrome, Cutler syndrome, **Herrmann syndrome,** MERRF syndrome, and Treft syndrome. However, the ophthalmic symptoms associated with Kearns-Sayre syndrome distinguish it from other mitochondrial disorders.

Keutel Syndrome

Also Known As: Pulmonic stenosis, brachytelephalangism, and calcification of cartilages

This is a very rare syndrome with voice and hearing disorders. Fewer than 20 cases have been documented. The effect on voice is related to calcification of the laryngeal cartilages that results in abnormal mobility and articulation of the laryngeal structures.

Major System(s) Affected: Craniofacial; respiratory; skeletal; cardiopulmonary; central nervous system.

Etiology: Autosomal recessive inheritance. The gene has not been mapped or identified.

Speech Disorders: Obligatory anterior articulation distortions and substitutions are likely related to maxillary hypoplasia and Class III malocclusion.

Feeding Disorders: Early failure-to-thrive may occur secondary to pulmonic stenosis and decreased vitality. However, in most cases, feeding is normal.

Hearing Disorders: Sensorineural hearing loss is common.

Voice Disorders: Voice is hoarse related to calcification of the laryngeal cartilages.

Resonance Disorders: Resonance is normal.

Language Disorders: Language is impaired in some cases secondary to cognitive impairment.

Other Clinical Features:

Craniofacial: maxillary hypoplasia; depressed nasal tip;

Respiratory: calcification of the larynx; calcification of the trachea;

Skeletal: short terminal phalanges of all digits; calcified rib cartilage;

Cardiopulmonary: pulmonic stenosis, heart anomalies;

Central nervous system: occasional cognitive impairment.

Natural History: So few cases have been reported that it is not possible to know the exact nature of the progression of the disorder. However, the calcification is probably mildly progressive.

Treatment Prognosis: Unknown.

Differential Diagnosis: Maxillary hypoplasia with a depressed nasal tip is common in **Binder syndrome.** However, patients with **Binder syndrome** do not have respiratory or cardiac anomalies. Anomalies of the trachea associated with maxillary hypoplasia and a short nose is seen in **Stickler syndrome,** but the cartilages in **Stickler syndrome** are too soft, rather than calcified.

K

Klippel-Trénaunay-Weber Syndrome

Also Known As: Angioosteohypertrophy syndrome; Klippel-Trénaunay syndrome

This syndrome was delineated nearly 100 years ago and represents an unusual constellation of vascular anomalies that include multiple angiomas of the oral structures, including the tongue, lips, gingiva, and palate.

Major System(s) Affected: Vascular; craniofacial/oral; limbs; genitourinary; hematologic; gastrointestinal; central nervous system.

Etiology: Autosomal dominant inheritance has been speculated. The gene has not been mapped or identified. Somatic mutation has not been ruled out.

Speech Disorders: Articulation is impaired by oral angiomas preventing normal lip and tongue placement. The errors are obligatory. Hypervascularity can also cause overgrowth of the face that results in malocclusion resulting in additional articulatory distortions.

Feeding Disorders: Feeding is normal in infancy. Later in life, chewing and food transport may be impaired by angiomatous growths in the oral cavity and on the palate.

Hearing Disorders: Hearing is normal.

Voice Disorders: Voice is normal. Hemangiomas of the larynx have not been noted.

Resonance Disorders: Resonance is normal.

Language Disorders: Language is impaired in the small percentage of patients who have cognitive impairment. Cognitive impairment is found most often in patients who have facial hemangiomas and port-wine stains of the facial skin.

Other Clinical Features:

> **Vascular:** multiple angiomas and hemangiomas of the skin, limbs, face, and viscera; cavernous hemangiomas;

Craniofacial/oral: oral angiomas (lips, tongue, gingiva, palate); facial hemangiomas; facial asymmetry with unilateral overgrowth; enlarged teeth and maxilla on affected side; premature dental development on affected side;

Limbs: severe distortion of digits, arms, legs related to hypervascularity; limb hypertrophy;

Genitourinary: renal hemangiomas; uterine hemangiomas; renal artery aneurysm; enlarged genitals;

Hematologic: Kasabach-Merritt thrombocytopenia;

Gastrointestinal: internal organ hemangiomas;

Central nervous system: occasional cognitive deficiency; occasional seizures.

Natural History: The vascular anomalies are present at birth, but their effects are progressive with growth.

Treatment Prognosis: The prognosis is good if the central nervous system is not involved. Surgery and interventional procedures such as selective embolization may be effective in some cases.

Differential Diagnosis: The unilateral facial overgrowth in Klippel-Trénaunay-Weber syndrome is similar to that seen in **Sturge-Weber syndrome** and **hemihypertrophy,** but these syndromes do not involve the same limb anomalies. Similar limb malformations may be found in **Maffucci syndrome.**

Kniest Syndrome

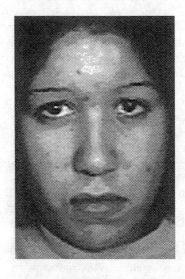

Characteristic facial appearance in Kniest syndrome.

Also Known As: Kniest dysplasia; metatropic dysplasia II; metatropic dwarfism, type II

Kniest dysplasia is one of the syndromes of short stature that is frequently associated with cleft palate. Clefting is found in over half the patients with Kniest syndrome. A number of genetic mutations in the same gene causes this skeletal dysplasia. **Stickler syndrome** and **spondyloepiphyseal dysplasia congenita** are caused by different sets of mutations in the same gene (COL2A1).

Major System(s) Affected: Growth; craniofacial; ocular; skeletal.

Etiology: Autosomal dominant inheritance. The gene has been mapped to the long arm of chromosome 12 and has been identified as a collagen 2 gene, COL2A1.

Speech Disorders: Children with Kniest syndrome may develop compensatory articulation patterns secondary to cleft palate and velopharyngeal insufficiency.

Feeding Disorders: Early feeding may be impaired by upper airway obstruction caused by micrognathia and Robin sequence. Resolution of the airway problems resolves the feeding disorder.

Hearing Disorders: Conductive hearing loss secondary to middle ear effusion is common. Approximately 15% to 25% of individuals with Kniest syndrome have sensorineural hearing loss, usually high frequency.

Voice Disorders: Voice may be mildly hoarse related to lax connective tissue in the larynx.

Resonance Disorders: Resonance may be hypernasal secondary to cleft palate.

Language Disorders: Language development is typically normal.

Other Clinical Features:

> **Growth:** short stature;

> **Craniofacial:** macrocephaly; maxillary and mandibular hypoplasia; round facies; depressed nasal root; Robin sequence;

> **Ocular:** myopia; tendency toward retinal detachment; strabismus; cataracts;

> **Skeletal:** flattened vertebrae (platyspondyly); thin joint spaces; joint limitation; joint enlargement; club foot; lordosis; odontoid hypoplasia leading to the risk of atlantoaxial instability.

Natural History: The skeletal dysplasia and short stature become evident in infancy. Robin sequence is possible, but does not occur with as high a frequency as in other COL2A1 disorders such as **Stickler syndrome** and **spondyloepiphyseal dysplasia congenita**. There is progressive deformation of the skeleton with age, including the potential for pulmonary restriction because of the spinal anomalies. Atlanto-axial instability may be present so that cervical spine radiographs need to be done and hyperextension of the neck avoided.

Treatment Prognosis: The skeletal dysplasia cannot be treated, but in general, the prognosis is good, including normal speech and language development.

Differential Diagnosis: Spondyloepiphyseal dysplasia congenita is another syndrome of short stature, Robin sequence, round facial appearance, and cleft palate. However, the radiographic findings are different and the type of X-ray findings are highly diagnostic of Kniest syndrome.

Laband Syndrome

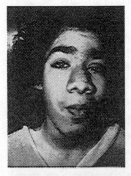
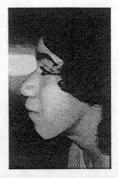

Prominent nose, thick lips, and absence of the terminal phalanges of the fingers in Laband syndrome.

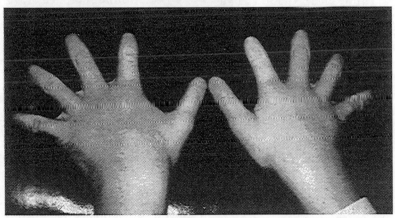

L

Also Known As: Zimmerman-Laband syndrome; gingival fibromatosis with abnormal fingers

Laband syndrome is a rare disorder, but it is easily recognized be-cause its constellation of clinical findings are distinctive. Most no-ticeable is the thickened alveolar ridges resulting from gingival fibromatosis. The fingers are also distinctive with the terminal phalanges missing in many cases.

257

Major System(s) Affected: Craniofacial/oral; limbs; gastrointestinal; central nervous system; integument.

Etiology: Autosomal dominant inheritance. The gene has not been mapped or identified.

Speech Disorders: Articulation is impaired by gingival overgrowth and the soft spongy texture of the maxillary alveolus. Dental eruption may be impaired because of the gingival overgrowth so that linguadental sound production is impaired.

Feeding Disorders: Feeding may be impaired by an inability to chew well because the gingival hyperplasia may cover the dentition.

Hearing Disorders: Hearing is typically normal.

Voice Disorders: Voice is typically normal.

Resonance Disorders: Resonance is typically normal.

Language Disorders: Language is impaired in cases with cognitive impairment.

Other Clinical Features:

Craniofacial/oral: gingival fibromatosis; large ears; large nose; large mouth; full lips; vertical facial growth pattern; steep mandibular plane angle;

Limbs: absence or hypoplasia of the terminal phalanges of the fingers and toes; dysplastic or absent nails;

Gastrointestinal: enlarged spleen; enlarged liver;

Central nervous system: occasional mental retardation or learning diabilities;

Integument: hirsutism.

Natural History: The gingival fibromatosis is present at birth, but does get progressively worse with time. The teeth erupt, but the continued overgrowth of the gingiva may result in little of the dentition being exposed above the gingival margin. With time, because of the alveolar overgrowth, the facial growth pattern becomes more vertical than normal, resulting in a steep mandibular plane angle.

Treatment Prognosis: The prognosis in general is good, with few limitations on the quality of life, but the gingival overgrowth is progressive.

Differential Diagnosis: There are a number of rare syndromes with gingival overgrowth, but the absence or hypoplasia of the terminal phalanges is distinctive in Laband syndrome. In addition, children who are treated with phenytoin for seizures may have gingival hyperplasia and cognitive impairment, as found in Laband syndrome. However, in the cases of phenytoin treatment, the effect is purely iatrogenic.

Langer-Giedion Syndrome

Also Known As: Trichorhino-phalangeal syndrome, Type II

Langer-Giedion is a well-recognized multiple anomaly syndrome that was initially grouped with another similar disorder, trichorhinophalangeal syndrome (now labeled trichorhinophalangeal syndrome type I), but was subsequently recognized to be a distinct and separate entity with some phenotypic overlap. It has since been found that Langer-Giedion syndrome is a contiguous gene disorder with the deletion from the long arm of chromosome 8 encompassing the single gene responsible for trichorhinophalangeal syndrome type I. Therefore, Langer-Giedion syndrome represents an expanded phenotype involving other genes surrounding the trichorhinophalangeal syndrome gene.

Major System(s) Affected: Skeletal; limbs; integument; craniofacial; central nervous system; genitourinary.

Etiology: Autosomal dominant inheritance. Langer-Giedion is caused by a contiguous gene deletion at 8q24.11-q24.13.

Speech Disorders: Speech is typically delayed disproportionate to the degree of cognitive impairment. There are no specific articulation disorders characteristic of the syndrome.

Feeding Disorders: Feeding in infancy is nearly a constant problem and is related to the combined effects of retrognathia and hypotonia.

Hearing Disorders: Sensorineural and mixed hearing loss occur in Langer-Giedion syndrome. The sensorineural component is progressive and moderate to severe in at least some cases.

Voice Disorders: Voice is typically normal.

Resonance Disorders: Resonance is normal.

Language Disorders: Language is delayed, especially in terms of expressive language.

Other Clinical Features:

Skeletal: multiple exostoses; hyperextensible joints; cone-shaped epiphyses in the hands;

Limbs: clinodactyly of the fingers;

Integument: sparse scalp hair; thick eyebrows; redundant skin;

Craniofacial: bulbous nose; broad nasal root; prominent philtrum; microcephaly; micrognathia;

Central nervous system: cognitive impairment; hypotonia;

Genitourinary: G-U reflux; persistent cloaca;

Other: prune belly.

Natural History: The diagnosis may be difficult at birth because of the absence of hair in many newborns. The skeletal and facial features become more pronounced with age. Feeding difficulties are common in infancy, but are not syndrome specific, nor are they different problems than found in other disorders with hypotonia and retrognathia.

Treatment Prognosis: Symptomatic treatment for the hearing and speech disorders is indicated and patients do respond to appropriate speech-language stimulation.

Differential Diagnosis: Trichorhinophalangeal syndrome type I shares many of the same phenotypic features as Langer-Giedion syndrome. The facial manifestations, hypotonia, and feeding difficulties in Langer-Giedion are similar to those found in **velocardio-facial syndrome,** but cleft palate is not a feature of Langer-Giedion.

Larsen Syndrome

Also Known As:

Larsen syndrome is a disorder of joint dislocations and cleft palate that has been reported to occur in two forms: autosomal recessive and autosomal dominant. The clinical presentation of the two forms are essentially the same, so they will be described as a single entry.

Major System(s) Affected:
Musculoskeletal; craniofacial; limbs.

Etiology:
The autosomal dominant form has been mapped to 3p21.1-014.1. The gene has been labeled LAR1. The autosomal recessive form has not been mapped. Although Larsen syndrome involves multiple joint dislocations, neither the dominant nor recessive forms have been linked to any of the collagen or fibrillin genes that have typically been associated with joint and skeletal abnormalities.

Speech Disorders:
Compensatory articulation patterns may occur secondary to cleft palate and velopharyngeal insufficiency.

Feeding Disorders:
Early feeding may be complicated by clefting, but is otherwise normal.

Hearing Disorders:
Conductive hearing loss occurs secondary to dislocations of the ossicles. Abnormalities of the footplate of the stapes also occur. Mixed and sensorineural hearing loss have been observed infrequently.

Voice Disorders:
Voice is normal.

Resonance Disorders:
Hypernasal resonance is common secondary to cleft palate.

Language Disorders:
Language and intellect are normal.

Other Clinical Features:

Musculoskeletal: multiple congenital joint dislocations; scoliosis;

Craniofacial: flattened midface; cleft palate;

Limbs: dislocation of the tibia; brachydactyly; extra carpal bones.

Natural History: The joint dislocations are present at birth and others may develop shortly after. Lax joints persist throughout life.

Treatment Prognosis: Surgical management is indicated for structural joint anomalies and palatal cleft. Intellect is normal.

Differential Diagnosis: Joint dislocations occur in **Hajdu-Cheney syndrome, otopalatodigidtal syndrome,** and Ehlers-Danlos syndrome. These syndromes have many other findings inconsistent with Larsen syndrome, including cognitive impairment (otopalatodigital), lax skin (Ehlers-Danlos), and dental anomalies (Hajdu-Cheney).

Laurence-Moon Syndrome

Also Known As:

Prior to the application of molecular genetics techniques, the association of obesity, pigmentary retinopathy, and mental retardation was classified as Laurence-Moon-Bardet-Biedl syndrome. It is now known, however, that all of the cases initially lumped together under Lawrence-Moon-Bardet-Biedl syndrome do not represent the same disorder. Four subtypes of Bardet-Biedl syndrome and Lawrence-Moon syndrome have now been recognized as distinct syndromes. Laurence-Moon differs phenotypically from the Bardet-Biedl syndromes by the absence of polydactyly and the presence of spastic paraplegia. The recessive genes for the Bardet-Biedl syndromes have been mapped, but the gene for Laurence-Moon syndrome is not yet known. All of these disorders have mental retardation as a constant finding.

Major System(s) Affected: Central nervous system; endocrine/growth; ocular; genitourinary.

Etiology: Autosomal recessive mode of inheritance. The gene has not yet been mapped.

Speech Disorders: Speech is typically very delayed, and in the most severe cases, speech may be very limited. Severe hypotonia may further impair articulation development.

Feeding Disorders: Severe hypotonia may result in a weak suck in infancy.

Hearing Disorders: Hearing is not impaired.

Voice Disorders: Voice disorders have not been documented.

Resonance Disorders: Resonance is normal.

Language Disorders: Language is always impaired. There is always significant delay in the onset of language milestones, and language develops slowly.

Other Clinical Features:

Central nervous system:
mental retardation; hypotonia; spastic paraplegia;

Endocrine/growth: obesity;

Ocular: pigmentary retinopathy;

Genitourinary: micropenis; hypogonadism.

Natural History: The developmental impairment associated with Laurence-Moon syndrome is present from birth. The retinopathy is progressive with onset in childhood. Eventual blindness occurs in most patients.

Treatment Prognosis: The overall prognosis for improvement in cognitive development and language is poor. As visual impairment progresses, the cognitive impairments may be exacerbated. Mental retardation varies from mild to moderate.

Differential Diagnosis: There are other syndromes that have cognitive impairment, obesity, and hypotonia as features, including the **Bardet-Biedl syndromes** (types 1 through 4), **Prader-Willi syndrome,** and **Cohen syndrome.**

Lenz Syndrome

Also Known As: Lenz microphthalmia syndrome; Lenz dysplasia; microphthalmia with associated anomalies

Lenz syndrome is one of a number of multiple anomaly disorders that has the association of eye anomalies and mental retardation. This association is not a surprising one because the eyes are embryologically closely related to the brain and formation of the prosencephalon, or forebrain.

Major System(s) Affected: Ocular; central nervous system; limbs; craniofacial; dental; musculoskeletal; growth; cardiac; gastrointestinal; genitourinary.

Etiology: X-linked recessive inheritance. The gene has not been mapped or identified.

Speech Disorders: Speech is typically delayed secondary to cognitive impairment. Speech may also be impaired by the development of compensatory articulation secondary to cleft palate and velopharyngeal insufficiency. Micrognathia may also contribute to

placement errors and distortions. Some patients have mild dysarthria or dyspraxia. Dental anomalies, including missing teeth and abnormally positioned teeth are common in the syndrome, resulting in obligatory distortions or substitution.

Feeding Disorders: Early feeding is impaired by the combination of hypotonia, micrognathia, and cleft palate. Airway obstruction may occur intermittently. Growth typically lags behind but is not impaired by poor feeding. Lenz syndrome has a primary growth disorder as a component of the syndrome.

Hearing Disorders: Conductive hearing loss secondary to middle ear effusion is possible. A few cases have demonstrated a unilateral sensorineural hearing loss.

Voice Disorders: Voice disorders have not been observed or reported.

Resonance Disorders: Hypernasal resonance secondary to cleft palate and velopharyngeal insufficiency is common.

266

Language Disorders: Language impairment, both expressive and receptive, is common. In some severe cases, language may be very limited.

Other Clinical Features:

Ocular: microphthalmia or anophthalmia (may be unilateral or bilateral); ocular colobomas (iris, retina, optic nerve); microcornea; strabismus; nystagmus;

Central nervous system: cognitive impairment;

Limbs: preaxial polydactyly (duplicated thumb); syndactyly; clinodactyly; camptodactyly;

Craniofacial: microcephaly; upslanting eyes; cleft palate; occasional cleft lip; dysplastic, featureless ears; protuberant ears; micrognathia; Robin sequence;

Dental: congenitally missing teeth; malocclusion; abnormal position of the central incisors;

Musculoskeletal: narrow sloping shoulders; hypoplastic clavicles; kyphoscoliosis; lumbar lordosis; webbing of the neck; long, narrow chest;

Growth: small stature;

Cardiac: bicuspid aortic valve;

Gastrointestinal: imperforate anus;

Genitourinary: hypospadias; cryptorchidism; renal aplasia or hypoplasia; hydroureter.

Natural History: The anomalies associated with Lenz syndrome are static, and all are present at birth. Development is persistently delayed in most cases and cognitive impairment becomes evident early in life.

Treatment Prognosis: Prognosis is heavily dependent on the degree of cognitive impairment. There is a relationship between the degree of ocular anomalies, as well. The prognosis is poorer for cases with bilateral anophthalmia or microphthalmia.

Differential Diagnosis: Anophthalmia or microphthalmia may be a feature of **oculo-auriculo-vertebral sequence,** but ear anomalies, cervical spine anomalies, and mandibular malformations can differentiate these conditions. Ocular anomalies, ear anomalies, and imperforate anus are also found in **CHARGE association** and rubella embryopathy.

Lenz-Majewski Syndrome

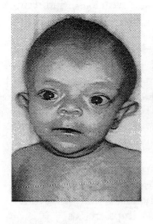
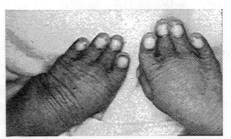

Characteristic facial appearance in Lenz-Majewski syndrome with associated digital anomalies including reduced length of the fingers.

Also Known As: Lenz-Majewski hyperostotic dwarfism

This unusual syndrome of short stature and mental retardation is rare, but distinctive. Most children with this syndrome are severely retarded.

Major System(s) Affected: Growth; craniofacial; limbs; musculoskeletal; central nervous system; dental; integument.

Etiology: Autosomal dominant expression is presumed, but has not been confirmed.

Speech Disorders: Speech does not develop in many patients, or is severely limited in others.

Feeding Disorders: Early feeding may be severely impaired because of upper airway obstruction related to choanal atresia.

Hearing Disorders: Sensorineural hearing loss is common.

Voice Disorders: Voice disorders have not been observed or reported.

Resonance Disorders: Resonance disorders have not been observed or reported.

L

Language Disorders: Language is severely impaired, and in some cases, little useful language is acquired.

Other Clinical Features:

Growth: short stature;

Craniofacial: orbital hypertelorism; large appearing neurocranium; prolonged patency of the fontanels; prominent scalp veins; large appearing mouth; choanal atresia;

Limbs: reduced finger length; hypoplastic long bones;

Musculoskeletal: rib and clavicular hyperostoses;

Central nervous system: mental retardation, often severe;

Dental: enamel hypoplasia;

Integument: loose, thin, wrinkled skin.

Natural History: Birth weight is low, and growth deficiency becomes progressive after birth. The head appears large in infancy. The fontanels remain patent into childhood. Developmental delay is obvious in infancy.

Treatment Prognosis: Poor because of irreversible nature of the skeletal dysplasia and the severity of cognitive impairment.

Differential Diagnosis: The large neurocranium and patent fontanels is similar to the craniofacial manifestations seen in **cleidocranial dysplasia**. The developmental delay in Lenz-Majewski syndrome is not consistent with the developmental pattern in **cleidocranial dysplasia**.

Lesch-Nyhan Syndrome

Also Known As: Hypoxanthine-guanine phosphoribosyltransferase deficiency

Lesch-Nyhan syndrome is rare (population frequency of approximately 1:100,000), but is one of the best known of genetic disorders because of the bizarre behavior of affected children, specifically self-mutilating biting of the lips and fingers resulting in disfiguring injuries. The syndrome is caused by a deficiency in the enzyme HPRT (hypoxanthine-guanine phosphoribosyltransferase deficiency).

Major System(s) Affected: Central nervous system; behavioral; genitourinary; hematologic.

Etiology: X-linked recessive inheritance. The gene, identified as HPRT, has been mapped to Xq26-q27.2. There are different mutations that all result in the disorder, including point mutations (base pair substitutions), deletions, and insertions.

Speech Disorders: Speech is marked by dysarthria, typically severe. In some cases, self-mutilation will result in severe injuries to the lips and tongue that will further interfere with articulation.

Feeding Disorders: Feeding disorders have not been associated with Lesch-Nyhan syndrome, in part because the onset of neurological symptoms occurs in childhood, not infancy. However, frequent vomiting is common in infancy, usually beginning by 6 months of age.

Hearing Disorders: Hearing loss has not been associated with Lesch-Nyhan syndrome.

Voice Disorders: Voice production is typically normal, but breath control and support may be poor.

Resonance Disorders: Resonance is abnormal secondary to dysarthria. Abnormal nasal and oral resonance occur.

Language Disorders: Language development is impaired and delayed, but most affected individuals do develop some expressive language.

L

Other Clinical Features:

Central nervous system: mental retardation, IQ ranging from 40 to 80; dysarthria; hyperreflexia; athetoid movements of the hands and feet; eventual choreiform movements; hypotonia in infancy followed by ataxia, chorea, and dystonia and then evolving to hypertonicity and spasticity;

Behavioral: self-mutilation, particularly biting of the lips, fingers, and hands; head banging; diminution of self-destructive behavior in adolescence;

Genitourinary: uric acid renal stones; obstructive nephropathy;

Hematologic: megaloblastic anemia;

Other: gout; hyperuricemia.

Natural History: Psychomotor development begins to slow and become obviously impaired in infancy, typically between 3 and 6 months of age. A slowing of growth is evident, as well. Self-mutilation begins in childhood, typically near the third birthday and usually begins with biting of the lips, cheeks, and tongue, later progressing to the fingers, hands, and arms. Head banging and compulsive rocking begin slightly later. The self-destructive behaviors begin to diminish in adolescence, but may be triggered by external events. Life expectancy is short, depending on management of the uric acid levels. Without treatment, death may occur in childhood, between 5 and 10 years of age. With treatment, death usually occurs before 20 years of age.

Treatment Prognosis: Very poor. There is no definitive treatment for the enzymatic deficiency and the self-mutilation. Therefore, restraints and mechanical devices to prevent self-mutilation provide the best option for the avoidance of injury. Uric acid abnormalities can be treated with allopurinol.

Differential Diagnosis: Self-mutilation may occur in a number of disorders that have congenital indifference to pain, but the overall developmental pattern and urinary excretion abnormalities associated with Lesch-Nyhan make the diagnosis easy to confirm.

Lowe Syndrome

Also Known As: Oculo-cerebro-renal syndrome

Lowe syndrome is a rare X-linked syndrome of mental retardation that has a number of ocular findings that complicate the clinical management of affected patients. Relatively few cases have been published in the literature, but it is likely that the syndrome is under-reported and not recognized frequently.

Major System(s) Affected: Central nervous system; ocular; skeletal; genitourinary.

Etiology: X-linked recessive inheritance. The gene has been mapped to Xq26.1. The gene has been labelled OCRL. A number of different mutations have been identified, all leading to the phenotype.

Speech Disorders: Speech onset is severely delayed and impaired. Some patients do not develop significant speech. In patients who do develop speech, there is severe neurologic impairment in most.

Feeding Disorders: Early failure-to-thrive is a common manifestation of the syndrome, secondary to severe hypotonia, chronic vomiting, and dehydration. Constipation is also common. Refusal to eat and anorexia have been observed.

Hearing Disorders: Hearing loss has not been reported or observed as a consistent feature of Lowe syndrome.

Voice Disorders: High-pitched screaming has been observed in many cases.

Resonance Disorders: Resonance disorders have not been reported as a consistent feature of Lowe syndrome.

Language Disorders: Language is consistently impaired, often severely, both receptively and expressively, with the delays commensurate to the cognitive impairment.

Other Clinical Features:

> **Central nervous system:** mental retardation; hypotonia in infancy; severe psychomotor delays and impair-

L

ments; reduced or absent deep tendon reflexes; tremors; aggressive and maladaptive behaviors;

Ocular: congenital cataracts; nystagmus; enophthalmus; glaucoma; corneal scarring;

Skeletal: vitamin D resistant rickets; joint hyperextensibility;

Genitourinary: cryptorchidism; renal failure.

Natural History: Many babies with Lowe syndrome appear normal at birth, but expression of the developmental and psychomotor disorders becomes obvious during infancy. The disorder becomes progressive with time. Chronic renal failure may lead to death in childhood.

Treatment Prognosis: Very poor. There is no definitive treatment for Lowe syndrome. Palliative treatment involving the use of Vitamin D, ophthalmologic treatment, and other supportive therapies may be useful, but progress with communicative disorders is slow because of the restrictions of severe retardation.

Differential Diagnosis: Cognitive impairment and ocular anomalies are common in fetal rubella embryopathy.

Maffucci Syndrome

Also Known As: Osteochondromatosis; enchondromatosis

Maffucci syndrome was initially described over 100 years ago. The disorder is rare, but very unusual in presentation and therefore easily diagnosed. The syndrome is distinguished by multiple tumors, starting with enchondromas, cartilaginous tumors, that are typically first established on the hands and feet.

Major System(s) Affected: Skeletal; integument; neoplastic.

Etiology: Unknown.

Speech Disorders: Speech development is typically normal, but speech production can be impaired by oral hemangiomas. Other neoplasias occur in the syndrome, including tumors of the head and neck that can interfere with jaw movement and articulation. Brain anomalies and neoplasias may also result in neurologic events that can interfere with speech production.

Feeding Disorders: Feeding is not usually impaired initially, but may be hindered by oral hemangiomas or other tumors that impinge on the airway.

Hearing Disorders: Hearing loss has not been associated with Maffucci syndrome.

Voice Disorders: Voice disorders have not been associated with Maffucci syndrome.

Resonance Disorders: Resonance disorders have not been associated with Maffucci syndrome.

Language Disorders: Language development is typically normal. Later in life, if brain tumors develop, language may be secondarily impaired.

Other Clinical Features:

Skeletal: osteochondromatosis; tubular bone abnormalities; enchondromas;

Integument: multiple hemangiomas, especially oral;

Neoplastic: chondrosarcomas; ovarian tumors; pancreatic carcinoma; pituitary tumors; brain tumors.

M

Natural History: Most patients are normal at birth. Hemangiomas usually appear first, often by the first birthday or shortly after. Enchondromas occur later in childhood or by adolescence. The enchondromas may lead to bone weakness and fracure in about one-quarter of cases. Cancerous changes occur later in life.

Treatment Prognosis: In cases where the growths are benign, surgical removal is possible. However, in some cases, the tumors are too widespread and difficult to remove. Some patients have undergone amputation.

Differential Diagnosis: Both **Klippel-Trénaunay-Weber syndrome** and **Proteus syndrome** have similar pervasive skin lesions, but only Maffucci syndrome has enchondromas.

Mannosidosis

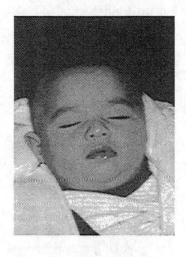

Mild coarsening of the face in an infant with mannosidosis.

Also Known As: Alpha-mannosidosis; alpha-mannosidase B deficiency

Mannosidosis is another of the lysosomal storage diseases, similar in some ways to **Hurler, Hunter, Sanfilippo,** and **Morquio syndromes.** As in other lysosomal disorders, absence of a particular enzyme (in this case alpha-mannosidase) prevents the degradation of glycoproteins in the intracellular structures known as lysosomes. The glycoproteins are stored in the cells, thus distorting the cells and their functions. As with other lysosomal disorders, there is more than one form of the disease, a severe form with early onset (type I) and a milder form with late onset (type II).

Major System(s) Affected: Growth; central nervous system; craniofacial; musculoskeletal; hematologic; respiratory; immunologic, ocular.

Etiology: Autosomal recessive inheritance. The gene has been mapped to chromosome 19, at 19cen-q12 (from the centromere to the q12 band on the long arm of chromsome 19).

Speech Disorders: Infants with type I do not develop speech. Individuals with type II have delayed onset of speech. They tend to have sluggish articulation secondary to macroglossia and cognitive impairment. Dental spacing problems also lead to articulatory distortions.

Feeding Disorders: Infants with type I have failure-to-thrive secondary to severe neurologic impairment and chronic upper airway obstruction. In type II, feeding may be complicated by chronic congestion.

Hearing Disorders: In type II, high-frequency sensorineural hearing loss is very common.

Voice Disorders: Voice is hoarse and wet secondary to chronic congestion and thickening of the vocal cord mucosa.

Resonance Disorders: Hyponasality is common secondary to chronic nasal congestion. The sensorineural hearing loss may contribute to the abnormal oral and nasal resonance patterns that accompany this type of hearing impairment.

Language Disorders: Infants with type I do not live long enough to develop language. In type II, language is essentially always delayed and impaired, but most individuals do obtain adequate language for communication.

Other Clinical Features:

Growth: tall stature;

Central nervous system: mental retardation; dilated ventricles; ataxia;

Craniofacial: coarse facial features; macrocephaly; thickened calvarium; low anterior hairline; thick, flat nose; macroglossia; gingival hypertrophy; mandibular prognathism; dental spacing; large, thick ears; bushy eyebrows;

Musculoskeletal: hypotonia; pectus carinatum; spondylosis;

Hematologic: abnormal lymphocytes; pancytopenia;

Respiratory: chronic upper and lower respiratory infections; chronic otitis;

Immunologic: immunoglobulin deficiency; hypogammaglobulinemia;

Ocular: corneal opacities.

Natural History: Newborns with type I do not survive infancy. The survival for type II is more favorable, but the onset of cognitive impairment and delayed development is early. The disorder is progressive, as are all lysosomal storage diseases.

Treatment Prognosis: Bone marrow transplantation has been suggested as being of possible benefit to patients with mannosidosis. However, no specific benefit of treatment has been demonstrated to date. Palliative treatment is certainly indicated.

Differential Diagnosis: Although the general features of all lysosomal storage diseases are similar, the diagnosis of the specific disorder is based on appropriate biochemical tests.

Marden-Walker Syndrome

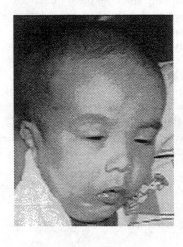

Lack of facial animation and extreme facial hypotomia in Marden-Walker syndrome.

Also Known As:

Marden-Walker is a rare, but probably under-reported, syndrome of mental retardation associated with cleft palate and Robin sequence. Failure-to-thrive is one of the key findings in this syndrome.

Major System(s) Affected:

Craniofacial; central nervous system; growth; gastrointestinal; musculoskeletal; renal; ocular.

Etiology:

Autosomal recessive inheritance. The gene has not been mapped or identified.

Speech Disorders:

Speech is always delayed, and in some cases, there is no significant speech development. In most cases, speech is very limited and marked by significant discoordination, dyspraxia, and dysarthria.

Feeding Disorders:

Early failure-to-thrive is one of the most common manifestations of the syndrome and has multiple causative contributions, including upper airway obstruction (micrognathia, hypotonia, Robin sequence), generalized hypotonia, and congenital heart anomalies. Cleft palate may further complicate early efforts at feeding.

Hearing Disorders: Hearing impairment has not been reported or observed, but mild conductive hearing loss secondary to middle ear disease should be anticipated in patients with cleft palate (approximately one-third of cases).

Voice Disorders: Voice disorders have not been reported or observed.

Resonance Disorders: Hypernasality secondary to the combined effects of cleft palate, hypotonia, and dysarthria should be anticipated.

Language Disorders: Language impairment is always present and is usually severe. There has not been a systematic study of language disorders in Marden-Walker syndrome.

Other Clinical Features:

Craniofacial: cleft palate; micrognathia; Robin sequence; microcephaly; hypertelorism; facial paresis or hypotonia;

Central nervous system: mental retardation, often severe; cerebellar hypoplasia; absent corpus callosum; hypoplastic brain stem; ventricular dilation; absent primitive reflexes; diminished deep tendon reflexes; hypotonia;

Growth: small stature;

Gastrointestinal: pyloric stenosis; pancreatic insufficiency;

Musculoskeletal: kyphoscoliosis; joint contractures; pectus excavatum or carinatum;

Renal: microcystic kidney disease;

Ocular: small eyes; ptosis.

Natural History: Developmental and neurological impairment is evident at birth. The absence of reflexes and hypotonia are sufficiently severe to be noticed even in the neonatal period. Failure-to-thrive is also obvious immediately. Developmental impairment is global.

Treatment Prognosis: The prognosis for significant rehabilitation is typically poor because of the severity of central nervous system malformation and dysfunction.

Differential Diagnosis: The severity of developmental delay associated with Robin sequence, joint contractures, and failure-to-thrive is found in Miller-Diecker syndrome (lissencephaly). Brain imaging will differentiate these disorders.

Marfan Syndrome

Also Known As:

Marfan syndrome is a well-recognized syndrome of connective tissue abnormalities that results in multiple skeletal and joint abnormalities. Marfan syndrome probably has a population prevalence of approximately 1:10,000.

Major System(s) Affected:
Musculoskeletal; ocular; craniofacial; cardiac; pulmonary.

Etiology: Autosomal dominant inheritance. Most cases are familial, but approximately 20% are new mutations. The gene has been mapped to 15q21.1 and has been identified as the fibrillin gene.

Speech Disorders: Articulation impairment is common secondary to malocclusion resulting in obligatory substitutions and distortions. Malocclusions typically involve vertical maxillary excess, maxillary constriction, dental crowding, and anterior skeletal open-bite. The dentofacial abnormalities are progressive. Therefore, articulation impairment often involves lingual protrusion.

Feeding Disorders: Feeding in infancy is usually normal. Later in life, malocclusion may lead to some chewing difficulties.

Hearing Disorders: Sensorineural hearing loss is not a common finding, but has been observed in some cases.

Voice Disorders: Hoarse voice is an occasional finding related to pulmonary disease.

Resonance Disorders: Resonance is typically normal.

Language Disorders: Language development is normal, as is cognition.

Other Clinical Features:

Musculoskeletal: tall, thin body with disproportionately long limbs (known as marfanoid habitus); scoliosis or kyphoscoliosis; pectus carinatum or excavatum; joint laxity; joint contractures; arachnodactyly;

Ocular: ectopia lentis (dislocated lens); myopia; retinal detachment;

Craniofacial: dolicocephaly; vertical maxillary excess with "long face"; anterior skeletal open-bite, vertical growth pattern; dental crowding;

Cardiac: aortic aneurysm; aortic dissection; aortic regurgitation; mitral valve prolapse; aortic root dilation; right-sided heart enlargement and congestive heart failure;

Pulmonary: restrictive pulmonary disease; emphysema; pneumothorax; pulmonary blebs.

Natural History: The facial and skeletal manifestations of Marfan syndrome are progressive, but typically become evident early in life. The cardiac and vascular anomalies may arise at any time, but sudden death secondary to aortic dissection is most common in early adult years. Early death is common. Cognition and overall development are normal.

Treatment Prognosis: Careful follow-up of cardiac status, especially aortic anomalies, is extremely important. Early management of scoliosis and spinal anomalies is also recommended to avoid pulmonary restriction. Increased intracardiac pressures can further exacerbate aortic dissections so that maintaining normal pulmonary capacity is important.

Differential Diagnosis: Joint hyperextensibility associated with myopia and "marfanoid habitus" may be observed in **Stickler syndrome.** Cleft palate, common in **Stickler syndrome,** does not occur in Marfan syndrome.

Marinesco-Sjögren Syndrome

Also Known As:

This is a rare syndrome with a direct impact on speech because of severe neurological problems leading to dysarthria and cognitive impairment.

Major System(s) Affected:
Central nervous system; ocular; growth; endocrine; musculoskeletal.

Etiology: Autosomal recessive inheritance.

Speech Disorders: Speech is typically delayed and articulation impaired by neurological disorders, most often involving moderate to severe dysarthria.

Feeding Disorders: Early feeding may be complicated by poor coordination and spasticity.

Hearing Disorders: Hearing loss has not been reported or observed.

Voice Disorders: Voice is characterized by poor breath control.

Resonance Disorders: Abnormal oral and nasal resonance secondary to dysarthria are common.

Language Disorders: Language delay and impairment are common. Most patients do develop some speech, but in severe cases of cognitive impairment, language development is very limited or absent.

Other Clinical Features:

Central nervous system: mental retardation; cerebellar ataxia; dysarthria; spasticity; cerebellar cortical atrophy; microcephaly;

Ocular: nystagmus; strabismus; congenital cataracts;

Growth: short stature;

Endocrine: hypergonadotropic hypogonadism;

Musculoskeletal: kyphoscoliosis; pectus carinatum; coxa valga; cubitus valgus; joint contractures; myopathy with elevated serum creatine kinase.

Natural History: All anomalies are present at birth and there is progression of neurologic symptoms.

Treatment Prognosis: Poor. Palliative treatment is indicated, but there will be severe limitations on progress with speech and language therapy.

Differential Diagnosis: The presence of congenital cataracts with progressive neurologic disease is found in a number of lysosomal storage diseases, but these may be ruled out with appropriate metabolic tests.

Maroteaux-Lamy Syndrome

Also Known As: Mucopolysaccharidosis type VI; arylsulfatase B deficiency

Maroteaux-Lamy syndrome has three subtypes: mild, moderate, and severe. In all three types, unlike many of the lysosomal storage diseases, cognitive abilities are normal in almost all cases. However, coarsening of the face and short stature are consistent findings. The syndrome is rare and does not occur more than 1:100,000 births.

Major System(s) Affected: Craniofacial; growth; ocular; cardiopulmonary; musculoskeletal; abdominal/gut.

Etiology: Autosomal recessive inheritance. The gene has been mapped to 5q11-q13.

Speech Disorders: Speech development is often normal initially, but articulation may often become impaired secondary to enlargement of the tongue and eventual malocclusion related to dental eruption problems secondary to thickened gingiva and alveolar bone abnormalities.

Feeding Disorders: Feeding is typically normal. Later in life, enlargement of the tongue and dental eruption abnormalities may cause some difficulty with chewing large or tough pieces of food.

Hearing Disorders: Both conductive and sensorineural hearing losses have been observed, but are not necessarily common manifestations of the syndrome.

Voice Disorders: Hoarseness is common secondary to mucosal thickening and chronic mucus buildup in the upper and lower airway.

Resonance Disorders: Resonance is initially normal, but with age and progression of the phenotype, hyponasality may occur secondary to chronic nasal congestion, especially in the most severe cases. Oral resonance may also be abnormal secondary to thickening of the tongue, oral mucosa, and tonsils.

Language Disorders: Language development is almost always normal.

Other Clinical Features:

Craniofacial: coarse facial appearance; enlarged tongue; thickened maxillary and mandibular alveolus; dental spacing anomalies; dental eruption anomalies; thickened palate and buccal surfaces; thickened mucosa;

Growth: short stature;

Ocular: corneal opacities;

Cardiopulmonary: valve anomalies; chronic upper and lower airway disease; pulmonary insufficiency;

Musculoskeletal: joint stiffness; lumbar kyphosis; genu valgum; hip dysplasia; pectus carinatum;

Abdominal/gut: inguinal hernia; hepatosplenomegaly.

Natural History: The age of onset varies for the three subtypes. In the mildest form, onset is usually in childhood at about school age, while in the milder form, onset is in infancy. In all subtypes, cognition is normal, but the other findings vary in severity.

Treatment Prognosis: There is no known treatment for the progressive nature of the anomalies. In the mildest form, patients survive to adult years. In the most severe form, premature death may occur in adolescence or late childhood caused by the combined effects of heart valve abnormalities and pulmonary disease.

Differential Diagnosis: The coarsening facial features and growth deficiency are near consistent findings in the majority of the lysosomal storage diseases. The differentiation is made by laboratory tests.

Marshall Syndrome

Also Known As:

Marshall syndrome is a disorder that has been regarded to be clinically similar to **Stickler syndrome,** and in the past, many clinicians believed that **Stickler syndrome** and Marshall syndrome were simply variable expressions of the same disorder. Some clinicians called both disorders the Marshall-Stickler syndrome. However, it now seems apparent that **Stickler syndrome** and Marshall syndrome are separate disorders with Stickler being a far more common form of connective tissues dysplasia.

Major System(s) Affected:
Craniofacial; integument; ocular.

Etiology: Autosomal dominant inheritance. The gene has been mapped to 1p21 and has been identified as a collagen gene, COL11A1.

Speech Disorders: Articulation may be impaired by malocclusion, including a Class II relationship with open-bite, and constriction of the maxillary arch. Compensatory articulation patterns occur second-ary to cleft palate and velopharyngeal insufficiency.

Feeding Disorders: Upper airway obstruction is a possible finding in Marshall syndrome that may interfere with infant feeding.

Hearing Disorders: Sensorineural hearing loss occurs in a high percentage of patients with Marshall syndrome. The loss is typically high frequency and may be progressive.

Voice Disorders: Voice is normal.

Resonance Disorders: Hypernasal resonance occurs in some cases with cleft palate. However, nasal obstruction secondary to a small nasal capsule and a small nasopharynx may also occur.

Language Disorders: Language and cognition are usually normal.

Other Clinical Features:

Craniofacial: maxillary deficiency; cleft palate; mild

micrognathia; hypertelorism; thickening of the neuro-cranium;

Integument: patches of cutis aplasia;

Ocular: high myopia; cataracts; glaucoma; strabismus; retinal detachment possible with age.

Natural History: At birth, some babies with Marshall syndrome present with Robin sequence, but this association is not as frequent as with **Stickler syndrome.** Midfacial deficiency becomes evident with age, but is not apparent in infancy. However, the malocclusion often remains Class II with a maxillary overjet because the mandible may be hypoplastic as well. Myopia is often present and severe at birth and becomes progressively worse with age. Hearing loss may be mildly progressive.

Treatment Prognosis: The prognosis is excellent. Cognition is normal. Myopia can be managed with spectacles and eventually with surgery, as can retinal detachment. Speech outcome from surgical repair of the palate is usually excellent.

Differential Diagnosis: Stickler syndrome has a very similar phenotype, but without the cutis aplasia or calvarial thickening. **Stickler syndrome** also has joint abnormalities and epiphyseal dysplasia.

Marshall-Smith Syndrome

Also Known As:

This is a rare syndrome, but one that presents with the usual association of accelerated growth in the presence of failure-to-thrive. Affected individuals rarely survive past 3 years of age.

Major System(s) Affected:
Craniofacial; central nervous system; growth; respiratory; skeletal.

Etiology: Unknown.

Speech Disorders: Speech does not develop secondary to severe cognitive impairment and shortened life span.

Feeding Disorders: Failure-to-thrive is a constant finding, but it is accompanied by advanced skeletal maturation and accelerated linear growth. Failure-to-thrive is a consequence of severe cognitive impairment, respiratory compromise, and hypotonia.

Hearing Disorders: Hearing disorders have not been reported or observed.

Voice Disorders: Crying is hoarse with inspiratory stridor.

Resonance Disorders: Not applicable (speech does not develop).

Language Disorders: There is no expressive language development, and little or no receptive language development.

Other Clinical Features:

Craniofacial: prominent, high forehead; short anterior cranial base; depressed nasal root; micrognathia; choanal atresia or stenosis;

Central nervous system: severe neurologic impairment; pachygyria;

Growth: early accelerated linear growth, but weight is disproportionately low compared to length;

Respiratory: severe respiratory and pulmonary compromise; chronic pneumonia;

Skeletal: advanced skeletal age;

Ocular: blue sclerae.

Natural History: Respiratory distress is evident shortly after birth and failure-to-thrive is immediate. Multiple pneumonias and pulmonary insufficiency are present in infancy and become progressively worse. Death usually occurs in infancy or early childhood secondary to respiratory compromise.

Treatment Prognosis: Very poor.

Differential Diagnosis: Accelerated growth is common in **Weaver syndrome** and **Sotos syndrome,** but without the severe respiratory complications and early death.

Mohr Syndrome

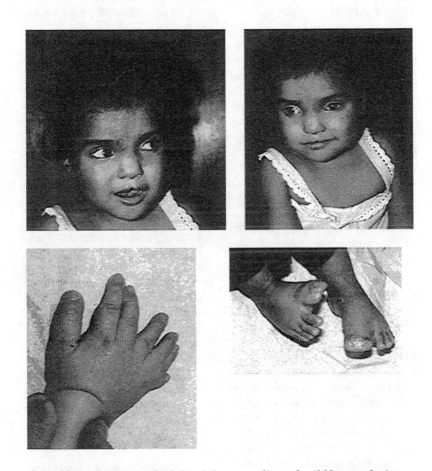

Central notching (pseudocleft) of the upper lip and mild hypertelorism (top row) associated with polydactyly in Mohr syndrome (OFD type II).

293

Also Known As: Oral-facial-digital syndrome, type II; OFD II

Mohr syndrome is one of the multiple anomaly disorders that have been classified as **oral-facial-digital syndromes.** The label oral-facial-digital does not connote any genetic or etiologic common ground, but rather is a descriptive nosological term based on several of the major clinical findings. The syndrome is rare with a population frequency of 1:300,000.

Major System(s) Affected: Craniofacial; growth; central nervous system; limbs.

Etiology: Autosomal recessive inheritance. The gene has not been mapped or identified.

Speech Disorders: Speech is delayed in many cases, especially those with more significant cognitive impairment. Articulation is typically impaired secondary to lingual abnormalities including a lobulated tongue and hamartomas of the tongue. A midline cleft of the lip also makes bilabial sound production difficult. Compensatory articulation patterns secondary to cleft palate and velopharyngeal insufficiency may also occur.

Feeding Disorders: Feeding may be complicated by newborn tachypnea.

Hearing Disorders: Conductive hearing loss secondary to ossicular malformation, particularly of the incus, is common.

Voice Disorders: Voice is typically normal.

Resonance Disorders: Hypernasal resonance secondary to cleft palate may occur.

Language Disorders: Language impairment is constant in patients with cognitive impairment and central nervous system anomalies. In the most severe cases, there is limited language development.

Other Clinical Features:

> **Craniofacial:** midline cleft lip; cleft palate; lobulated or cleft tongue; lingual hamartomas; abnormal cranial sutures;

> **Growth:** short stature;

> **Central nervous system:** cognitive impairment; cerebellar anomalies;

> **Limbs:** polydactyly; syndactyly.

Natural History: All of the anomalies associated with Mohr syndrome are present at birth and are essentially static.

Treatment Prognosis: The prognosis depends on the degree of cognitive impairment and CNS anomalies. Some individuals with Mohr syndrome have died in childhood secondary to respiratory infections.

Differential Diagnosis: Digital and craniofacial anomalies are common features in all of the **oral-facial-digital syndromes.** Midline cleft lip is common in the premaxilary agenesis type of **holoprosencephaly.**

M

Morquio Syndrome

Also Known As: Mucopolysaccharidosis type IV; galactosamine-6-sulfatase deficiency

Morquio syndrome is another autosomal recessive lysosomal storage disease with a progressive course, but longer survival than **Hunter, Hurler,** or **Sanfilippo syndrome.** Also somewhat different than the other mucopolysaccharidoses, there is little, if any, facial coarsening in Morquio syndrome, with more of the effects being seen in the extracranial skeleton. Two subtypes have been described, a severe form labeled as MPS IVA and a mild, late onset type labeled MPS IVB. However, individuals clinically diagnosed with MPS IVB do not have galactosamine-6-sulfatase deficiency, indicating that the disorder is etiologically and genetically different than classic Morquio syndrome.

Major System(s) Affected: Growth; musculoskeletal; ocular; gastrointestinal; cardiopulmonary.

Etiology: Autosomal recessive inheritance. The gene has been mapped to 16q24.3 and has been labeled GALNS.

Speech Disorders: Speech is essentially normal, but there is relative prognathism in some cases that may result in distortion of anterior sound production.

Feeding Disorders: Feeding is typically normal.

Hearing Disorders: Conductive hearing loss secondary to chronic middle ear effusion and "glue ear" is common.

Voice Disorders: Voice is typically high-pitched and hoarse in adolescent and adult years.

Resonance Disorders: There is an unusual oropharyngeal resonance related to a short neck and limited resonating cavity. In adult years, persistent hyponasality is common secondary to chronic nasal congestion and obstruction.

Language Disorders: Language development and intellect are normal.

Other Clinical Features:

Growth: short stature (average adult height is approximately 3 feet);

Musculoskeletal: kyphoscoliosis; hip dysplasia; pectus carinatum; platyspondyly (flat vertebrae); antlanto-axial instability caused by a hypoplastic odontoid process that may result in spinal cord and nerve compression; joint laxity; genu valgum; thickened calvarial bones; increased space between the vertebrae; wide metaphyses; osteoporosis;

Ocular: corneal opacities;

Gastrointestinal: inguinal hernias; umbilical hernia; liver enlargement;

Cardiopulmonary: valve anomalies; aortic regurgitation; restrictive pulmonary disease (secondary to skeletal anomalies).

Natural History: The onset of noticeable physical findings in Morquio syndrome is at approximately 2 years. Progression of respiratory symptoms and hearing loss is relatively slow compared to other lysosomal storage diseases. Most patients live into adult years, usually to the 20s or 30s, but complications of pulmonary restriction and possible spinal injury can complicate the prognosis and cause earlier death.

Treatment Prognosis: The long-term prognosis is poor, but palliative treatment in early life for middle ear disease is effective.

Differential Diagnosis: Morquio syndrome does not have the same facial phenotype as the other mucopolysaccharidoses, but the extracranial findings are similar. Also, unlike other mucopolysaccharidoses, intellect and behavior are normal. Severe kyphoscoliosis and short stature are common in diastrophic dysplasia and flattened vertebrae may be found in **spondyloepiphyseal dysplasia congenita.** However, the overall pattern of skeletal dysplasias in these syndromes is different and there are no signs of metabolic disease as in Morquio syndrome.

Multiple Lentigines Syndrome

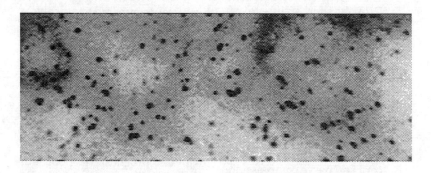

Appearance of the skin, Multiple letigines syndrome, showing multiple lentigines, small darkly pigmented growths.

Also Known As: LEOPARD syndrome; lentiginosis, cardiomyopathy

This syndrome was first identified as LEOPARD syndrome, an acronym for multiple *L*entigines, *E*lectrocardiographic conduction abnormalities, *O*cular hypertelorism, *P*ulmonic stenosis, *A*bnormal genitalia, *R*etarded growth, and sensorineural *D*eafness. The acronym is an attempt at humor because dark lentigines are distributed in many places on the body making individuals appear spotted like a leopard. Cutaneous abnormalities associated with cognitive impairments and hearing loss are common among other syndromes (such as neurofibromatosis and basal cell nevus syndrome), so that obvious pigmentary abnormalities should always raise an index of suspicion with the observant clinician.

Major System(s) Affected: Integument; cardiopulmonary; genitourinary; growth/endocrine; craniofacial.

Etiology: Autosomal dominant inheritance. The gene has not been mapped or identified.

Speech Disorders: Speech and articulation are typically normal. However, there have been a number of cases with relatively large growths on the hard or soft palate that could interfere with tongue placement for articulation. In cases with severe or profound hearing loss (unusual), speech production will be severely impaired.

Feeding Disorders: Feeding is normal.

Hearing Disorders: Mild sensorineural hearing loss is a common, but not consistent feature of the syndrome. Several cases have been known to have more severe hearing loss. Vestibular abnormalities have not been found.

Voice Disorders: Voice production is normal.

Resonance Disorders: Resonance abnormalities have not been reported or observed except in relation to sensorineural deafness.

Language Disorders: Language is mildly impaired in many cases secondary to cognitive impairment.

Other Clinical Features:

Integument: multiple small lentigines on the skin, not the mucous membranes; café-au-lait spots; occasional neoplasias;

Cardiopulmonary: valvular pulmonic stenosis; cardiomyopathy; ECG abnormalities;

Genitourinary: hypoplastic/aplastic ovaries; cryptorchidism; hypospadias;

Growth/endocrine: short stature; late onset of puberty;

Craniofacial: ocular hypertelorism.

Natural History: The lentigines are typically present at birth and increase in number with age. The heart and hearing anomalies may not be obvious at birth, but are present at birth. Growth deficiency is of postnatal onset.

Treatment Prognosis: All disorders can be treated symptomatically with the prognosis being based on the severity.

Differential Diagnosis: Basal cell nevus syndrome has a similar appearance of the skin, but the other anomalies are not similar. The association of the heart and genitourinary problems make this diagnosis distinctive.

Nager Syndrome

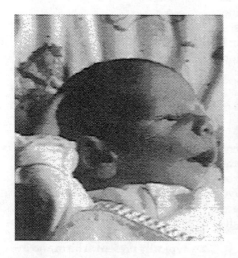 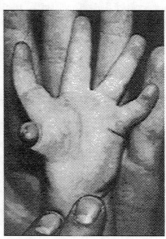

Severe micrognathia, Robin sequence, and hypoplasia of the thumb in an infant with Nager syndrome.

Also Known As: Acrofacial dysostosis; acrofacial dysostosis 1, Nager type; preaxial acrofacial dysostosis

Nager syndrome is a rare craniofacial disorder that closely resembles **Treacher Collins syndrome,** but has the added finding of radial and hand anomalies. The syndrome has some striking findings, including severe micrognathia and severe hypoplasia of the soft palate. The author has seen several cases with lit-

tle more than a uvula extending from the hard palate.

Major System(s) Affected: Craniofacial; limbs.

Etiology: The etiology of Nager syndrome has been debated since the disorder was first recognized. Autosomal recessive and autosomal dominant inheritance have both been proposed, but the majority of cases have been sporadic. Recessive inheritance seems likely with several instances of affected siblings with normal parents having been observed. Etiologic heterogeneity has not been ruled out.

Speech Disorders: Articulation disorders are a near constant in Nager syndrome. Unusually severe micrognathia leads to Class II occlusal relationships, open-bite, and limited oral opening. The tongue is often quite small, but still has difficulty maneuvering in a small oral cavity. Tongue-backing is a common articulatory maneuver leading to very abnormal substitutions that are probably obligatory in nature. Cleft palate is common, and the cleft is often very severe, resulting in compensatory patterns that include tongue backing, glottal stops, pharyngeal stops, and laryngeal stops.

Feeding Disorders: Early failure-to-thrive secondary to airway obstruction is very common. Tracheotomy is often necessary in Nager syndrome because of the severity of micrognathia. Robin sequence is a common secondary disorder in Nager syndrome.

Hearing Disorders: Conductive hearing loss is a near constant finding with ossicular malformations,

variable microtia, and fixation of the footplate of the stapes.

Voice Disorders: Voice is typically normal.

Resonance Disorders: Resonance is almost always anomalous with abnormalities of both oral and nasal resonance. Nasal resonance may be either hyponasal (if the palate is intact) or hypernasal (if the palate is cleft). In some cases, there is mixed hyper-hyponasality. Some patients with clefts have almost no soft palate with the uvula extending off of the hard palate with little intervening tissue. In such cases, palate reconstruction becomes extremely difficult and may require pharyngeal flap. However, because of the potential for airway obstruction, pharyngeal flap may not be possible without some advancement of the mandible. Oral resonance is usually very muffled because of posterior positioning of the tongue. In cases where the palate is cleft, the combination of muffled oral resonance with velopharyngeal insufficiency yields a very abnormal and unusual resonance pattern.

Language Disorders: Language development is typically

normal and intellect is typically normal.

Other Clinical Features:

Craniofacial: micrognathia, usually severe; cleft palate; microtia; ossicular anomalies; downslanting eyes; lower lid depressions; absent eyelashes of the inner third of the eye; zygomatic hypoplasia or clefting; acute flexion of the cranial base;

Limbs: radial hypoplasia; absent or hypoplastic thumbs; radio-ulnar synsotosis; decreased extension of elbows.

Natural History: All of the anomalies associated with Nager syndrome are present at birth and are nonprogressive. A pectus excavatum may develop because of upper airway obstruction resulting in negative pressure and rib cage distortion. There is no "catch-up" growth of the mandible with age.

Treatment Prognosis: The severity of the craniofacial anomalies in Nager syndrome make early reconstruction difficult. The severe deficiency of tissue in the palate will often prevent early palate repair. Mandibular distraction may have significant advantages in Nager syndrome because of the severity of the mandibular deficiency. Because failure-to-thrive is related to airway obstruction, treatment of obstructive apnea should be aggressive prior to recommending alternative feeding procedures.

Differential Diagnosis: Nager syndrome is almost identical to **Treacher Collins syndrome** in relation to the craniofacial findings, but **Treacher Collins syndrome** does not have limb anomalies as a clinical finding.

Neurofibromatosis, Type 1

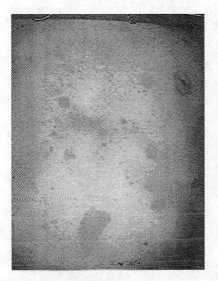
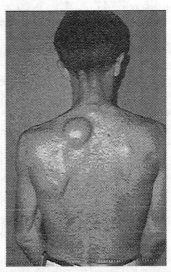

Neurofibromatosis type I (von Recklinghausen): Early presentation showing multiple café-au-lait spots on the skin of the abdomen and chest (left). Large neurofibroma in an adult.

Also Known As: von Recklinghausen disease; NF1; neurofibromatosis, von Recklinghausen type

Neurofibromatosis, type 1, is a common genetic disorder with a high spontaneous mutation rate. The disorder is known to be caused by a single gene mutation with a population prevalence of approximately 1:4,000. It is now known that there are at least nine distinct disorders that have been previously lumped under the title of neurofibromatosis, including NF1. Acoustic neuroma is not a feature of NF1, but is a major finding in NF2.

Major System(s) Affected: Integument; craniofacial; central nervous system; ocular; skeletal; cardiac.

Etiology: Autosomal dominant inheritance. The gene has been mapped to 17q11.2 and has been sequenced. The NF1 gene is large with approximately 60 exons and a size of 350 kilobases (350,000 base pairs). Over 180 separate mutations have been identified that result in NF1. Mutations include deletions, insertions, and point mutations. Approximately half of all cases are caused by new mutations.

Speech Disorders: Speech onset is often delayed. Mild dysarthria has been observed. Impaired articulation secondary to malocclusion is also found.

Feeding Disorders: Feeding disorders have not been a common observation.

Hearing Disorders: Hearing is typically normal in NF1.

Voice Disorders: Hoarseness secondary to asymmetry of the vocal cords has been observed.

Resonance Disorders: Hypernasality secondary to asymmetric movement of the velopharyngeal valve has been observed and reported.

Language Disorders: Language delay and impairment is common. Expressive language may be more severely impaired than receptive in some cases.

Other Clinical Features:

Integument: multiple café-au-lait macules located all over the body, but with the fewest on the face and increased freckling near the arm pits and groin; eventual development of a variety of tumors that may be distributed on the face;

Craniofacial: facial tumors; facial asymmetry; macrocephaly; oral tumors; malocclusion related to skeletal asymmetry of the mandible and/or maxilla;

Central nervous system: macrencephaly; learning disorders; seizures; occasional mental retardation; hydrocephaly; neuronal heterotopia;

Ocular: optic nerve glioma; Lisch nodules; glaucoma; ptosis; corneal opacity;

Skeletal: scoliosis;

Cardiac: pulmonary stenosis; supravalvular aortic stenosis; other heart anomalies (low frequency);

Other: various tumors may develop, including some malignancies.

Natural History: At birth, there may be no sign of anomalies. Usually the first presentation is the café-au-lait macules with tumors developing later in life. Life expectancy may be decreased in some cases secondary to tumor formation, occasional malignancy, or complications from benign growths. In some cases, there is developmental delay and learning impairment. Language is often affected, as is speech production. However, speech disorders can respond to standard treatments unless related to the presence of a CNS lesion or structural oral anomaly. In most cases when speech and language disorders are detected in young children, tumors are not at the root of the problem.

Treatment Prognosis: Fair to excellent depending on the type and location of tumors.

Differential Diagnosis: Café-au-lait spots may be found in over 100 genetic disorders. Abnormal tumor and hamartoma growth occurs in **Proteus syndrome, Bannayan-Zonana syndrome,** and **Klippel-Trénaunay-Weber syndrome.** Asymmetric craniofacial growth is found in **hemihyperplasia** and McCune-Albright syndrome.

N

Niikawa-Kuroki Syndrome

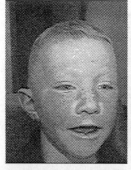
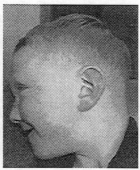
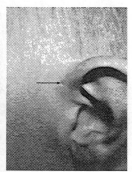

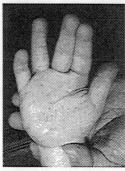

Note the wide palpebral fissures, large ears, preauricular pit (arrow at far right), and thickened finger pads in Niikawa-Kuroki syndrome.

Also Known As: Kabuki syndrome; Kabuki makeup syndrome

Niikawa-Kuroki syndrome is most often referred to as Kabuki syndrome, a name initially coined based on facial appearance. The appearance of the eyes with eversion of the lateral portion of the lids showing the red conjunctiva gave the impression of the makeup worn by Kabuki theater performers in Japan. The use of the term "Kabuki," although not specifically meant to be humorous, has a connotation that can be interpreted as being pejorative because of the exaggerated makeup style of Kabuki performers. It is therefore preferred to use the eponym of Niikawa-Kuroki syndrome in honor of the scientists who initially described the syndrome. The incidence of the syndrome is not known in all populations, but an estimated 1:30,000 individuals are affected in Japan. The syndrome is probably equally common worldwide.

Major System(s) Affected: Craniofacial; central nervous system; growth; cardiac; limbs; musculoskeletal.

Etiology: Autosomal dominant inheritance. The gene has not been mapped or identified.

Speech Disorders: Many children with Kabuki syndrome develop only limited speech. Others have severe articulatory impairment related to cognitive impairment and hypotonia, as well as the secondary effects of cleft palate and velopharyngeal insufficiency leading to compensatory articulation.

Feeding Disorders: Early feeding is often problematic based on multiple causes. Congenital heart anomalies (often severe) and hypotonia (often severe) lead to early failure-to-thrive and may result in the use of alternative feeding procedures, such as gavage feedings or gastrostomy.

Hearing Disorders: Conductive hearing loss is common in infancy and childhood secondary to chronic otitis media. Malformed ossicles may also be found.

Voice Disorders: Voice may be hoarse or high pitched.

Resonance Disorders: Hypernasal resonance is common in cases with cleft palate which may, in part, be related to the hypotonia common in the syndrome.

Language Disorders: Language is essentially always impaired, and often severely impaired. The onset of first words is severely delayed in most cases, and other language milestones are also very delayed.

Other Clinical Features:

Craniofacial: wide palpebral fissures; everted lateral portions of the lower eyelids with conjunctival show; microcephaly; cleft palate; large ears with prominent ear lobes; open-mouth posture; wide nose with depressed nasal tip;

Central nervous system: mental retardation; seizures;

Growth: small stature;

Cardiac: conotruncal heart anomalies; aortic aneurysm; right bundle branch block; transposition of the great vessels; single ventricle;

Limbs: persistent fetal finger pads;

Musculoskeletal: scoliosis; spina bifida occulta; abnormal hip joints; rib anomalies.

Natural History: Early neonatal course is difficult because of the combined effects of congenital heart disease, hypotonia, and neurologically based developmental impairment, and failure-to-thrive. Language milestones tend to be delayed and impaired more significantly than cognitive performance might predict. Small stature becomes apparent in infancy with postnatal growth deficiency.

Treatment Prognosis: Variable, depending on the degree of cognitive impairment. Although language and speech milestones seem to be disproportionately affected, treatment should be implemented as soon as possible and as vigorously as possible.

Differential Diagnosis: The association of conotruncal heart anomalies with cleft palate and hypotonia is common in **velo-cardiofacial syndrome** (VCFS). However, in VCFS, the ears are small with overfolded helices and absent lobules, whereas in Niikawa-Kuroki syndrome, the ears are large and the lobule prominent. Small stature, heart anomalies, and cleft palate may also be found in **fetal alcohol syndrome** (FAS), but in FAS, the palpebral fissures are short and the ears tend to be small.

Noonan Syndrome

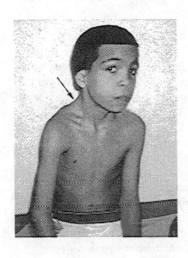

Note pterygium coli (arrow) and low set, posteriorly rotated ears in Noonan syndrome.

Also Known As: Pterygium coli syndrome

Noonan syndrome is a disorder that bears a strong physical resemblance to Turner syndrome, but is not associated with a sex chromosome abnormality and is not limited to expression in females. It is one of the more common multiple anomaly syndromes with a population prevalence of approximately 1:2500.

Major System(s) Affected: Craniofacial/head and neck; cardiac; central nervous system; growth; genitourinary; musculoskeletal; hematologic; integument.

Etiology: Autosomal dominant inheritance. The gene has been mapped to 12q24.

Speech Disorders: Speech is marked by many obligatory articulation errors related to malocclusion, including class II malocclusion, anterior skeletal open-bite, and a constricted maxillary arch. There is, in some patients, limitation of mandibular movement secondary to vertical maxillary excess and a steep mandibular plane an-

N

gle. Cleft palate is a low-frequency anomaly, and in most cases is submucous when present. Submucous cleft may lead to compensatory articulation patterns secondary to velopharyngeal insufficiency.

Feeding Disorders: Early feeding problems and failure-to-thrive are common problems, occurring in nearly half of cases. Feeding is complicated by airway obstruction, or by congenital heart disease, particularly pulmonary stenosis. Hypotonia is also present in approximately one third of cases.

Hearing Disorders: Conductive, sensorineural, and mixed hearing loss have all been observed in Noonan syndrome, but are relatively low-frequency anomalies.

Voice Disorders: Voice is typically normal, but in some cases with more severe growth deficiency, it may be high-pitched.

Resonance Disorders: Resonance may be hypernasal in a small percentage of patients with Noonan syndrome secondary to cleft palate (usually submucous). Oral resonance is occasionally muffled because the neck may be shorter than normal reducing the resonating volume of the oropharynx and hypopharynx.

Language Disorders: Language development is variable and is dependent on the presence of cognitive impairment. Intellect in Noonan syndrome ranges from mild mental retardation to superior intelligence, with approximately a third of cases showing some cognitive impairment. Language delay is common and has been attributed to perceptual-motor problems. Expressive language is usually proportionately more impaired than receptive. Learning disabilities have also been noted.

Other Clinical Features:

Craniofacial/head and neck: webbing of the neck (pterygium coli); cervical hygroma; triangular facial contour; deep furrow in the philtrum; prominent cupid's bow; vertical maxillary excess; vertical facial growth pattern with steep mandibular plane; low-set ears; posteriorly rotated ears; low posterior hairline; ptosis; mild orbital hypertelorism, downslanting eyes; anterior skeletal open-bite; constricted maxillary arch;

Cardiac: pulmonary stenosis; pulmonary valve dysplasia; patent ductus arteriosus; coarctation of the aorta; cardiomyopathy;

Central nervous system: cognitive impairment; perceptual impairments; learning disabilities;

Growth: short stature;

Genitourinary: cryptorchidism; male infertility;

Musculoskeletal: pectus excavatum and/or carinatum; "shield-shaped" chest; cubitus valgus; short distal phalanges;

Hematologic/lymphatic: lymphedema; von Willebrand disease; thrombocytopenia;

Integument: cutaneous lymphangioma; tendency toward easy bruising;

Other: malignant schwannoma.

Natural History: Developmental delay is relatively mild in cases with cognitive impairment, but in those cases, speech tends to be disproportionately delayed and expressive language more significantly impaired than intellect would predict. Thrombocytopenia may not be noted until later in life. Lymphedema may be present early, and may even be detected prenatally using ultrasound. If the heart anomalies are not too severe, life expectancy may be normal, although some patients do develop malignancies. Some patients with severe heart anomalies have a shortened life span.

Treatment Prognosis: The prognosis for Noonan syndrome is dependent on the severity of the heart anomalies and cognitive status. In general, the speech, language, and learning disorders do respond favorably to traditional therapeutic approaches. The facial anomalies and malocclusion typically require surgical intervention in teen years. Therefore, speech therapy, although effective for the language disorders and speech delay, will have little or no impact on obligatory sound errors caused by malocclusion.

Differential Diagnosis: Webbing of the neck is common in

Turner syndrome, but all Turner cases are phenotypically female and have an obvious karyotypic abnormality. The Noonan phenotype has also been observed in patients with **velo-cardio-facial syndrome,** including webbing of the neck, cryptorchidism, learning disabilities, thrombocytopenia, pulmonary stenosis, short distal phalanges, and disproportionately delayed expressive language. However, learning and cognitive problems are more common in VCFS, and mental illness is a manifestation of VCFS that has not been reported as a manifestation of Noonan syndrome.

Oculo-Auriculo-Vertebral Dysplasia (or Spectrum)

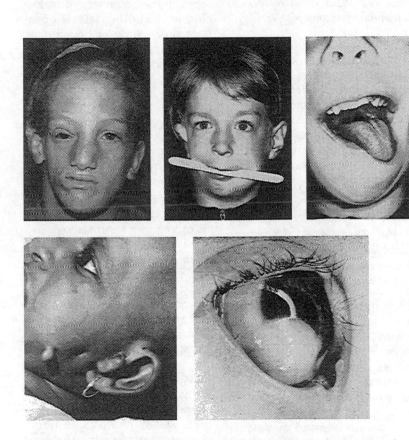

Oculo-auriculo-vertebral dysplasia: Note facial asymmetry, upward cant of the bite plane and asymmetric tongue movement (top row), ear tags and pits, and ocular dermoid (bottom row).

Also Known As: Hemifacial microsomia; facio-auriculo-vertebral sequence; lateral facial dysplasia; Goldenhar syndrome; OAVS

Oculo-auriculo-vertebral dysplasia (OAVS) is one of the most common craniofacial anomalies in man, perhaps second only to cleft palate as a type of craniofacial malformation. The population prevalence of the disorder is approximately 1:5,000. It is probable that an infant born with unilateral microtia has OAVS, unless the microtia is a feature of another syndrome such as **Treacher Collins syndrome.**

Major System(s) Affected: Craniofacial; ocular; musculoskeletal; central nervous system, cardiopulmonary.

Etiology: OAVS is etiologically heterogeneous. The disorder is not a specific syndrome, per se, but rather a developmental sequence that is presumed related to an embryonic vascular disruption in many cases. However, OAVS does occur as a secondary sequence in other syndromes and malformation sequences, including trisomy 18, del(18q), and velo-cardio-facial syndrome.

Speech Disorders: Speech is delayed in many cases. Articula-

tion impairment is very common with obligatory distortions and substitutions secondary to malocclusion, including lateral open-bites, anterior skeletal open-bites, micrognathia (unilateral or bilateral), unilateral paresis of the tongue and/or face; and missing dentition. Unilateral facial nerve paresis is common. Unilateral macrostomia is also common and may result in some distortions of sounds produced in the front of the oral cavity. Cleft lip and alveolus, a common malformation associated with OAVS, will also cause placement errors and distortions. Ankyloglossia caused by a short genioglossus muscle (often unilaterally) is also common. Compensatory articulation patterns secondary to cleft palate and velopharyngeal insufficiency are also common. Glossoptosis resulting in upper airway obstruction often results in fronting errors with lingual protrusion.

Feeding Disorders: Early feeding is frequently impaired and failure-to-thrive is a common early manifestation of OAVS. In nearly all cases, early feeding problems are related to airway obstruction. Unilateral hypoplasia of the pharynx and micrognathia combined with ankyloglossia results in upper airway obstruction and difficulty in coordinating breathing and eating. Many babies burn enormous amounts of calories just maintaining respiration and lose weight. When older, dental and occlusal anomalies may make chewing certain foods difficult. Feeding may also be complicated by some of the associated anomalies occasionally found in OAVS, including congenital heart disease, tracheoesophageal fistula, anal malformations, and pulmonary anomalies.

Hearing Disorders: Conductive hearing loss, usually unilateral, is a near constant finding. Middle and external ear malformations may range from fixation of the footplate of the stapes to complete absence of the external and middle ear. Many cases of OAVS have bilateral manifestations so that conductive hearing loss may be bilateral, but asymmetric. Sensorineural components to the hearing loss have been observed in a small percentage of cases, including some cases with complete agenesis of the inner ear.

Voice Disorders: Hoarse or breathy voice secondary to unilateral vocal cord paresis is a common finding.

Resonance Disorders: Hypernasal resonance secondary to cleft palate is common, but hypernasality is also observed secondary to unilateral paresis and hypoplasia of the palate and/or pharynx. Asymmetric velopharyngeal insufficiency is a common manifestation of the syndrome and is actually more common than central velopharyngeal gaps even in cases with cleft palate.

Language Disorders: Language development is typically normal, unless one of the associated findings is cognitive impairment. In some cases, cognitive impairment is severe and language does not develop, but these are unusual cases and are typically part of another syndrome complex that has OAVS as a secondary sequence.

Other Clinical Features:

Craniofacial: unilateral or bilateral hypoplasia of the mandible; absence of the condyle and/or coronoid (unilateral); absence or hypoplasia of the ramus (unilateral); facial nerve paresis; micrognathia; cleft palate; cleft lip and alveolus; preauricular skin tags and/or pits; cervical skin tags; microtia; anotia; ossicular malformations or aplasia; absence of the glenoid fossa (unilateral); macrostomia; lateral oral commissue cleft; cleft or absence of the zygoma (unilateral); lateral or anterior skeletal open-bite; shifting malocclusions; asymmetric movement of the palate and pharynx; unilateral hypoplasia of the pharynx or palate; hypoplasia or aplasia of the parotid glands; asymmetric cranium;

Ocular: clefts of the eyelids or orbits; microphthalmia; anophthalmia; dermoid cysts of the conjunctiva or limbus; orbital dystopia; strabismus;

Musculoskeletal: cervical spine anomalies; vertebral fusions; occipitalization of the atlas; Klippel-Feil anomaly; hemivertebrae; butterfly vertebrae; spina bifida occulta; scoliosis; rib anomalies; club foot; occasional limb anomalies including thumb and radial malformations;

Central nervous system: occasional cognitive impairment; encephalocele; brain lipoma; Arnold-Chiari anomaly; holoprosencephaly; arachnoid cyst;

Cardiopulmonary: various heart malformations, including ventriculoseptal defect, tetralogy of Fallot, atrial septal defect; aplastic or hypoplastic lungs.

Natural History: Many infants with OAVS have severe airway obstruction at birth that may require tracheotomy. Failure-to-thrive should be a strong indication that airway obstruction is occurring, and prior to implementing operative approaches to feeding disorders (i.e., gastrostomy), the approach should be to resolve the airway obstruction. Tracheotomy is necessary in some cases. Conductive hearing loss is present from birth and hearing should therefore be assessed at the first possible sign of external ear anomalies or facial asymmetry. Cervical spine anomalies are also common and should be assessed immediately because hyperextension of the neck could result in damage to the spinal cord. Facial form and symmetry may be relatively normal at birth in milder cases, but with growth, the hypoplastic side becomes progressively smaller relative to the normal growing side. An upward cant to the bite plane develops and the occlusion may become unstable and shift because the lower arch does not match the upper arch. Compensatory downward overgrowth of the maxillary alveolus occurs on the side of the mandibular hypoplasia resulting in the canting of the bite plane. In the early teen years, the facial asymmetry becomes more pronounced because the normal side of the mandible undergoes its normal growth spurt while the hypoplastic side continues to lag.

Treatment Prognosis: In the absence of cognitive impairment, the prognosis is excellent because of the availability of excellent reconstructive procedures for the facial skeleton, the external ear, and the middle ear. Because the hearing loss is nearly always purely conductive, amplification can be successful in bringing hearing to normal limits if there is bilateral loss, and with unilateral hearing loss, most affected individuals function very well with preferential seating in school. New reconstructive procedures, such as osseous distraction, can have a positive outcome in relation to facial asymmetry and airway obstruction.

Differential Diagnosis: Facial asymmetry with ear tags occurs in Townes-Brocks syndrome (commonly) and **velo-cardio-facial syndrome** (uncommonly). **BOR (branchi-oto-renal syndrome)** has the association of preauricular ear pits, dysmorphic ears, and hearing loss. Microtia, usually bilateral, with conductive hearing loss, cleft palate, occasional cleft lip, respiratory disorders, failure-to-thrive, and micrognathia occurs in both **Treacher Collins syndrome** and **Nager syndrome,** and on occasion, these disorders can have mild facial asymmetry or ear tags. Cervical spine radiographs are certainly indicated when microtia occurs to help confirm the diagnosis with the added advantage of demonstrating potentially dangerous malformations of the cervical spine.

Oculocerebrocutaneous Syndrome

Also Known As: Delleman syndrome; OCCS

Oculocerebrocutaneous syndrome, or OCCS, is a rare disorder with varying types of cerebral malformation associated with skin lesions and eye anomalies, usually eyelid clefts. Some degree of facial and somatic asymmetry has been found in some cases.

Major System(s) Affected: Central nervous system; ocular; craniofacial; integument.

Etiology: Autosomal dominant expression is likely, but the gene has not been mapped or identified.

Speech Disorders: In many, if not most cases, significant speech does not develop.

Feeding Disorders: Early feeding may be impaired by severe neurologic deficits.

Hearing Disorders: Hearing disorders have not been reported or observed.

Voice Disorders: Voice disorders have not been reported or observed.

Resonance Disorders: Resonance disorders have not been reported or observed.

Language Disorders: Language impairment is typically severe and many, if not most children, do not develop significant or functional language.

Other Clinical Features:

> **Central nervous system:** cerebral anomalies including agenesis of the corpus callosum and cystlike spaces in the brain; Dandy-Walker anomaly; mental retardation, often severe;

> **Ocular:** cysts; microphthalmia; hamartomas;

> **Craniofacial:** clefts of the eyelids; skin tags on the face and near the orbits; craniofacial asymmetry;

Integument: focal dermal hypoplasia or aplasia; punch-like defects of the skin on and around the nose.

Natural History: The ocular and dermal lesions are evident at birth. Developmental delay is global and also evident shortly after birth. Some cases of OCCS have had more normal neurologic development with mild mental retardation.

Treatment Prognosis: For most cases, the prognosis is poor because of major brain malformations.

Differential Diagnosis: The presence of skin tags together with facial asymmetry is a common association with **oculo-auriculo-vertebral dysplasia.** However, the skin tags in OCC are located in the periorbital area, atypical for patients with OAV.

Oculo-Dento-Digital Syndrome

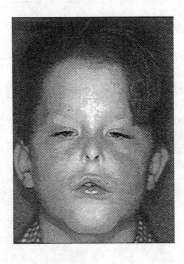

Oculo-dento-digital syndrome: Note the nasal alar hypoplasia.

Also Known As: Oculodentoosseous syndrome; oculodentodigital dysplasia; ODD

Oculo-dento-digital syndrome (ODD) is a rare autosomal dominant disorder with a high spontaneous mutation rate. The combination of ocular, dental, and hand anomalies is distinctive and easily recognized. Performance and cognitive abilities are typically normal.

Major System(s) Affected: Ocular; dental; craniofacial; limbs; integument; neurologic.

Etiology: Autosomal dominant inheritance. The gene has been mapped to 6q22-q24.

Speech Disorders: Articulation impairment is a common manifestation of ODD secondary to small teeth and dental gaps in both the maxillary and mandibular arches. Compensatory articulation secondary to cleft palate and velopharyngeal insufficiency is possible in some cases.

Feeding Disorders: Feeding disorders have not typically been associated with ODD.

Hearing Disorders: Conductive hearing loss has been found in some cases.

Voice Disorders: Voice is normal in ODD.

Resonance Disorders: Hypernasality secondary to cleft palate and hypernasality is a possible finding in some cases.

Language Disorders: Language development is normal.

Other Clinical Features:

Ocular: short palpebral fissure resulting in small-appearing eyes; microcornea; glaucoma;

Dental: small teeth; enamel hypoplasia;

Craniofacial: occasional cleft palate plus/minus cleft lip; small nose with hypoplastic alar rims; cranial hyperostoses; mandibular prognathism; hypotelorism;

Limbs: contractures of the fifth fingers; syndactyly of the ring finger and little finger and of the third and fourth toes; hypoplasia or aplasia of the middle phalanges, especially of the toes;

Integument: deficient scalp hair;

Neurologic: Spastic paraplegia and quadraplegia have been observed in a small number of cases; white matter hyperintensities on magnetic resonance imaging.

Natural History: The structural anomalies associated with ODD are present at birth except for the dental anomalies, which do not become apparent until dental eruption. Developmental milestones are normal and longevity is not affected. In cases with neurologic deficits, the quadraplegia or paraplegia have been progressive.

Treatment Prognosis: Dental anomalies can be treated effectively with bonding or implant procedures. Hypernasality and articulation disorders can be resolved after physical anomalies have been reconstructed. The neurologic disorders seen in some cases must be treated with palliative procedures, such as bracing.

Differential Diagnosis: The eye anomalies combined with the dental malformations in ODD are essentially unique.

Oculopharyngeal Muscular Dystrophy

Also Known As:

This autosomal dominant form of muscular dystrophy is particularly important in relation to speech production because of its specific effects on velopharyngeal function and swallowing. The syndrome has variable population frequency, apparently being more common in French Canadians from Quebec and Jews from Uzbekistan than in other populations. However, the disorder does occur in all racial and ethnic groups.

Major System(s) Affected: Ocular; neuromuscular.

Etiology: Autosomal dominant inheritance. The gene has been mapped to 14q11.2-q13 and has been identified as a gene encoding for the poly(A)-binding protein-2 (PABP2).

Speech Disorders: Speech is characterized by progressively sluggish articulation without significant dysarthria, but slowed by significant nasal air loss and an inability to impound oral pressure.

Feeding Disorders: Dysphagia is progressive and marked by some nasal regurgitation, and premature spillage from the oral cavity into the glottis because of poor or absent pharyngeal motility with absence of pharyngeal constriction during swallowing. However, glottic response is typically normal so that aspiration is not typical.

Hearing Disorders: Hearing is typically normal.

Voice Disorders: Voice is weak, primarily related to an inability to focus laryngeal vibrations by pharyngeal resonance.

Resonance Disorders: Severe hypernasality is the ultimate outcome of speech, starting with mild and progressive velopharyngeal insufficiency and nasal air escape with hypernasal resonance.

Language Disorders: Language development is normal.

Other Clinical Features:

Ocular: Progressive ptosis with weakening of the eyelids; pigmentary changes of the retina;

Neuromuscular: progressive pharyngeal paresis; eventual weakness of the facial, limb, and neck muscles.

Natural History: Individuals are normal at birth, but the disorder progresses once onset occurs. Onset is typically in the third decade of life, but this is variable.

Treatment Prognosis: There is no definitive treatment for the primary cellular defect. However, both hypernasality and ptosis can be treated surgically with proper anesthetic approaches. It is usually preferable to treat affected individuals initially with speech bulb prostheses because the initial degree of movement of the velopharyngeal muscles is likely to worsen with time. Therefore, treating the velopharyngeal insufficiency based on its initial presentation may not effectively anticipate the eventual status of the velopharyngeal valve.

Differential Diagnosis: Other muscular dystrophies also present with hypernasality, including facioscapulo-humoral muscular dystrophy and **Steinert syndrome** (myotonic dystrophy). However, these other disorders have other neuromuscular effects and earlier onset that oculopharyngeal muscular dystrophy.

Opitz Syndrome

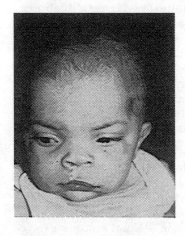

Opitz syndrome: Note hypertelorism.

Also Known As: G syndrome; BBB syndrome; G/BBB syndrome; Opitz-Frias syndrome; hypospadias-dysphagia syndrome; hypertelorism-hypospadias syndrome

Opitz syndrome has been the focus of some recent attention because of some clinical overlap between it and **velo-cardio-facial syndrome.** The clinical overlap between these two conditions has led some to believe that Opitz syndrome is also caused by a deletion of multiple genes at 22q11.2. However, the condition initially described by Opitz is clearly X-linked and does not resemble **velo-cardio-facial syndrome** at all. Cases with hypertel-orism and hypospadias that are deleted at 22q11.2 have **velo-cardio-facial syndrome,** not Opitz syndrome. The problem is not one of genetic heterogeneity, but rather one of diagnostic accuracy.

Major System(s) Affected: Craniofacial; genitourinary; gastrointestinal; central nervous system; cardiac.

Etiology: X-linked recessive inheritance. The gene has been mapped to Xp22 and has been labeled OSX.

Speech Disorders: Speech onset is typically delayed and articulation may be neurologically impaired. Cleft palate plus/minus cleft lip often results in compensatory articulation patterns secondary to velopharyngeal insufficiency.

Feeding Disorders: Early feeding is almost always impaired with aspiration secondary to laryngo-tracheoesophageal cleft. Hypotonia also complicates matters and may lead to upper airway obstruction. Esophageal dismotility has been reported, but is a presumptive diagnosis. Gastroesophageal reflux has also been observed.

Hearing Disorders: Conductive hearing loss secondary to chronic fluid and middle ear effusion is common.

Voice Disorders: Hoarse and/or breathy voice are common manifestations of the laryngotracheal clefts associated with Opitz syndrome.

Resonance Disorders: Hypernasality secondary to cleft palate and velopharyngeal insufficiency is common.

Language Disorders: Language is typically delayed and significantly impaired commensurate with cognitive deficiency. Cognitive impairment with mild to moderate mental retardation is a common, but not constant feature.

Other Clinical Features:

Craniofacial: hypertelorism; cleft palate plus/minus cleft lip; ankyloglossia;

Genitourinary: hypospadias; small male genitalia; bifid scrotum; renal or ureteral anomalies;

Gastrointestinal: laryngo-tracheoesophageal cleft; occasional imperforate anus; umbilical hernia;

Central nervous system: cognitive impairment; agenesis of the corpus callosum;

Cardiac: coarctation of the aorta; atrial septal defect.

Natural History: The initial presentation of the syndrome is a weak cry and aspiration during feeding secondary to the laryngeal cleft. Hypotonia and developmental delay becomes apparent, when present, in infancy. The genital hypoplasia and anomalies are also present at birth. Development is globally delayed in those cases with cognitive deficiency.

Treatment Prognosis: The prognosis is variable, depending on the presence of cognitive impairment and central nervous system anomalies. Reconstruction of the laryngeal cleft becomes necessary, but tracheotomy is obviously necessary in many cases until reconstruction has been complete.

Differential Diagnosis: Velo-cardio-facial syndrome has many of the same phenotypic features as Opitz syndrome, including hypospadias, occasional mild hypertelorism, cleft palate, developmental delay, hoarse voice (secondary to paresis or laryngeal web), hypotonia, and congenital heart anomalies. However, the appearance of the ears, nose, and digits is different than that seen in Opitz syndrome.

Oral-Facial-Digital Syndrome

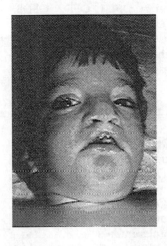
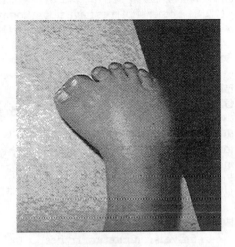

Oral-facial-digital syndrome: Note the cleft lip and palate associated with preaxial and postaxial polydactyly of the foot.

Also Known As: OFD

The oral-facial-digital syndromes are a group of eight separate disorders, each with a different genetic cause, but grouped together under the nosologic category of OFD because of the similarities in phenotypic expression, particularly in relation to the lobulated tongue and multiple oral frenula. For the sake of convenience, all of the disorders are listed under this single entry with each subtype's genotype and phenotype listed separately except for Mohr syndrome, which is listed separately under that commonly used heading.

Major System(s) Affected: Craniofacial/oral (all subtypes); limbs (all subtypes); integument (OFD1), central nervous system (all subtypes except OFD5), renal (OFD7).

Etiology: OFD1 and OFD8 are both X-linked recessive. OFD 3, OFD4, OFD5, and OFD6 are all autosomal recessive. OFD7 is probably autosomal dominant. OFD1 has been mapped to Xp22.3-p22.2. The other subtypes have not been mapped.

Speech Disorders: All of the oral-facial-digital syndromes are marked by significant speech delay. OFD1 is distinguished by eventual dysarthria. All of the oral-facial-digital syndromes have articulatory impairment related to abnormal tongue anatomy and the presence of hyperplastic oral frenulae.

Feeding Disorders: Early failure-to-thrive is common in all types of OFD except OFD5 secondary to cognitive impairment and central nervous system malformations. A substantial number of patients with OFD do not survive infancy.

Hearing Disorders: Conductive hearing loss has been demonstrated and observed in OFD1 and OFD4.

Voice Disorders: Voice disorders have not been observed in the oral-facial-digital syndromes.

Resonance Disorders: Hypernasality secondary to cleft palate may occur in OFD1, OFD4, and OFD6.

Language Disorders: Language impairment, often severe, is common in OFD1, OFD2, OFD3, OFD4, OFD6, OFD7, and OFD8. In the most severe cases, there is essentially no functional language development.

Other Clinical Features:

>   **Craniofacial/oral:** midline cleft or notch of the upper lip (OFD1, OFD5, OFD7); cleft lip plus/minus cleft palate (OFD4, OFD6, OFD8); lobulated tongue, hyperplastic oral frenulae;
>
>   **Limbs:** polydactyly;
>
>   **Integument:** multiple milia along the ears (OFD1);
>
>   **Central nervous system:** absence of the corpus callosum; porencephaly; cognitive impairment (all subtypes except OFD5);
>
>   **Renal:** kidney dysfunction (OFD7).

Natural History: All anomalies are present at birth. With the exception of OFD5, there is a high probability of marked delay of psychomotor development.

Treatment Prognosis: Prognosis is dependent on the degree of cognitive impairment. The digital and tongue anomalies can be managed surgically.

Differential Diagnosis: The challenge with the oral-facial-digital syndromes is distinguishing each from the other, in large part because of the need to provide appropriate genetic counseling.

Otopalatodigital Syndrome, Type 1

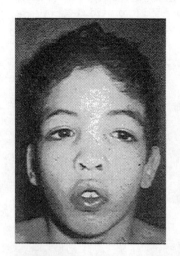
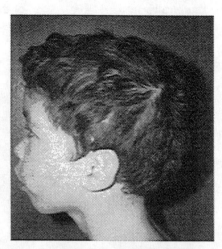

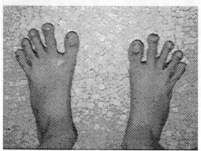
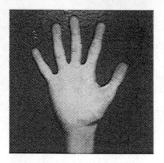

Otopalatodigital syndrome: Note the mild hypertelorism, downslanting palpebral fissures, and micrognathia (top row). The toes show shortened halluces and thickened finger pads with curved digits (bottom row).

Also Known As: OPD1

Otopalatodigital syndrome is a syndrome of cleft palate, micrognathia, and digital anomalies that also has the Robin sequence as an associated finding. The digit anomalies are distinctive. Although there are nosologically two forms of otopalatodigital syndrome and both are X-linked, there is little similarity between the two conditions in that the facial and digital anomalies are distinctively different between the two. Female heterozygotes tend to show minor manifestations of the gene, including minor digital anomalies.

Major System(s) Affected: Craniofacial; limbs; auditory; central nervous system; dental, growth.

Etiology: X-linked recessive inheritance. The gene has been mapped to Xq28.

Speech Disorders: Speech is typically delayed, usually mildly. Eventually speech is marked by articulation impairment related to malocclusion, including anterior skeletal open-bite. Tongue-backing is also common because of micrognathia and occasional ankyloglossia. Compensatory articulation disorders secondary to cleft palate and velopharyngeal insufficiency is common.

Feeding Disorders: Early failure-to-thrive is common and is almost always related to airway obstruction. Airway obstruction is prompted by the combination of micrognathia, an acute cranial base angle, and hypotonia. Resolution of the airway compromise will resolve the feeding problems.

Hearing Disorders: Conductive hearing loss is common and is related to both ossicular anomalies and chronic middle ear effusion.

Voice Disorders: Voice is typically normal.

Resonance Disorders: Cleft palate is a very common finding in the syndrome so that hypernasal speech is common.

Language Disorders: Language delay is a near constant finding with expressive language being somewhat more severely impaired than receptive. The degree of language involvement may be more significant than cognitive impairment would predict. Many cases have low normal intelligence, and most are borderline or have mild mental retardation.

Other Clinical Features:

Craniofacial: micrognathia; "pugilistic facies" with prominent brow and frontal bossing; broad nasal root; hypertelorism; downslanting eyes; downslanting oral commissures; acute cranial base angle;

Limbs: short halluces; widely spaced toes; clinodactyly; thick finger and toe pads; radial head dislocation; broad thumbs; short fingernails;

Skeletal: osteochondrodysplasia; scoliosis; pectus excavatum secondary to airway obstruction;

Auditory: conductive hearing loss;

Central nervous system: cognitive impairment;

Dental: hypodontia;

Growth: small stature.

Natural History: The digital anomalies may be difficult to recognize at birth and in infancy, as are the facial anomalies. The first signs of the syndrome may be cleft palate and failure-to-thrive. With age, the digital anomalies become more obvious and they are very distinctive in appearance.

Treatment Prognosis: The prognosis is typically good with speech and language disorders being amenable to therapy. Hearing disorders require amplification.

Differential Diagnosis: Digital, cleft, and micrognathia are common in **otopalatodigital syndrome, type 2** (OPD2), and **Nager syndrome,** but the distinctive appearance of the toes and fingers in OPD1 leaves little room for confusion.

Otopalatodigital Syndrome, Type 2

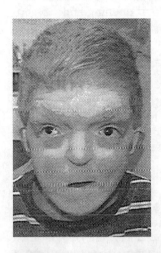
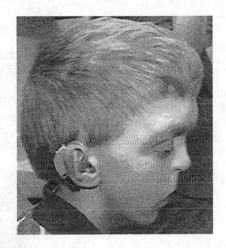

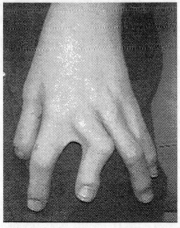

*Otopalatodigital syndrome type 2:
Note the hypertelorism and
micrognathia associated with
syndactyly and contractures.*

Also Known As: OPD2; cranio-orodigital syndrome

OPD2 is a rare syndrome that has been recognized infrequently and may be under-reported or diagnosed as another entity. The phenotype is more severe than OPD1 and actually does not resemble it particularly except for the groupings of anomaly types. Although both syndromes have limb anomalies, the anomalies are not similar.

Major System(s) Affected: Craniofacial; limbs; skeletal; genitourinary; abdominal; central nervous system.

Etiology: X-linked recessive.

Speech Disorders: Speech is marked by severe articulation impairment including retraction of all articulation in the posterior portion of the oral cavity because the entire oropharyngeal cavity is extremely small, including the mouth. The tongue is small, as is the mandible. Lingual protrusion is difficult and there may be significant ankyloglossia. Articulation is often in the floor of the mouth with poor tongue movement within the maxillary arch.

Feeding Disorders: Early failure-to-thrive and feeding disorders are common secondary to upper airway obstruction. There is very limited oral opening and glossoptosis. Aggressive management of the airway problems is recommended prior to alternative approaches to feeding.

Hearing Disorders: Conductive hearing loss secondary to ossicular malformations and fusions have been observed.

Voice Disorders: Voice is normal.

Resonance Disorders: Resonance is a mix of hypernasality (secondary to cleft palate) and muffled oral resonance (secondary to a small oropharynx and oral cavity). Although velopharyngeal insufficiency is common, the airway below the velopharyngeal valve is so limited in size even in rest position that the disordered resonance balance may be more severely impaired in the oral cavity than in the nasal cavity.

Language Disorders: Language development is often normal, but some cases have had hydrocephalus and secondary effects on the central nervous system. Cognitive impairment has been observed in some cases. Language impairment is commensurate to the degree of cognitive involvement.

Other Clinical Features:

Craniofacial: maxillary and mandibular hypoplasia; small mouth; cleft palate; down-turned oral commissures; hypertelorism; downslanting eyes; broad, high forehead;

Limbs: syndactyly; contractures; clinodactyly; bowing of the limbs; limitation of joint extension; absent fibula;

Skeletal: narrow chest;

Genitourinary: hypospadias; hydronephrosis; hydroureter;

Abdominal: omphalocele;

Central nervous system: hydrocephalus; occasional cognitive impairment.

Natural History: All anomalies are present at birth. Hydrocephalus may be called to attention in infancy secondary to abnormal head shape and head circumference. Airway obstruction and failure-to-thrive are common in infancy.

Treatment Prognosis: The prognosis is, in part, dependent on the presence or absence of central nervous system involvement. Skeletal structures can be managed surgically in many cases, including the hypoplasia of the mandible. Mandibular distraction may have a place in the management of the facial skeleton.

Differential Diagnosis: OPD1 has craniofacial and digital anomalies but without the broader spectrum of skeletal malformations. The craniofacial features in OPD2 are somewhat reminiscent of syndromes of craniosynostosis.

Pena-Shokeir Syndrome

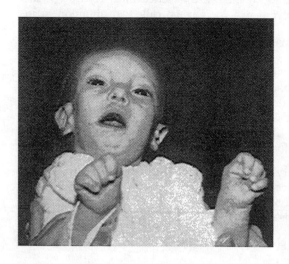

Note contractures in this infant with Pena-Shokeir syndrome.

Also Known As: Pena-Shokeir syndrome, type 1; fetal akinesia sequence

Although initially thought to be a specific syndrome, this disorder is now known to be an etiologically nonspecific developmental sequence, much like Robin sequence. Following the identification of Pena-Shokeir, a second similar disorder was delineated and initially labeled Pena-Shokeir, type 2. However, this second disorder, now referred to as COFS, or cerebrooculofacioskeletal syndrome (see entry in this text) is an autosomal recessive syndrome of known etiology. The disorder is important to recognize because it is relatively common (approximately 1:10,000 births) and presents with severe neonatal feeding problems.

Major System(s) Affected: Musculoskeletal; cardiopulmonary; central nervous system; craniofacial; limbs; integument; endocrine; genitourinary; gastrointestinal.

Etiology: Etiologically heterogenous. The disorder is related to

336

a lack of embryonic and fetal movement.

Speech Disorders: Speech does not develop. Many cases are stillborn, and most others die in the neonatal or infant period.

Feeding Disorders: There is severe failure-to-thrive, muscle wasting, upper airway obstruction, Robin sequence, and both upper and lower airway problems.

Hearing Disorders: Hearing data are not available.

Voice Disorders: Cry is weak, in part related to pulmonary hypoplasia.

Resonance Disorders: Not applicable.

Language Disorders: Language does not develop.

Other Clinical Features:

> **Musculoskeletal:** arthrogryposis and multiple joint contractures; muscle atrophy; hip and knee ankyosis; neck and axillary pterygia;

> **Cardiopulmonary:** pulmonary hypoplasia; small heart, congenital heart anomalies; arrhythmias;

> **Central nervous system:** deficiency of anterior horn cells in the spinal cord; primary motor neuropathy;

> **Craniofacial:** cleft palate; micrognathia; hypertelorism; microcephaly;

> **Limbs:** rocker-bottom feet; polydactyly; camptodactyly;

> **Integument:** scalp edema;

> **Endocrine:** adrenal hypoplasia;

> **Genitourinary:** cryptorchidism; hypospadias;

> **Gastrointestinal:** Meckel diverticulum.

Natural History: Infants with this disorder are small at birth and have immediate respiratory difficulties. A very high percentage die in the neonatal period, often of respiratory insufficiency and cardiac sequelae.

Treatment Prognosis: Extremely poor. Attempts to feed orally will always meet with failure and should be avoided.

P

Differential Diagnosis: Multiple joint contractures are found in arthrogryposis multiplex congenita and COFS. However, the pulmonary and cardiac hypoplasia are unique to Pena-Shokeir.

Pfeiffer Syndrome

Also Known As: Pfeiffer, type 1; acrocephalosyndactyly, type V

Pfeiffer syndrome is one of the well-recognized syndromes of craniosynostosis. Three subtypes of the disorder are now recognized. Pfeiffer syndrome, type 1 is the classically described phenotype of craniosynostosis and broad thumbs. In type 2, the disorder is characterized by cloverleaf skull, or kleeblattschädel, and limitation of movement at the elbows. Pfeiffer syndrome, type 3 has abnormalities of the gut and viscera in association with craniosynostosis and severe shortening of the anterior cranial base. Types 2 and 3 are fatal in infancy.

Major System(s) Affected: Craniofacial; limbs, central nervous system.

Etiology: Autosomal dominant inheritance. The gene has been mapped to two different loci. One mutation occurs in fibroblast growth factor receptor 2 (FGFR2), mapped to 10q26. The other mutation is in fibroblast growth factor receptor 1, mapped to 8p11.2-p11.1. Type 2 and type 3 forms of the disorder have more severe craniofacial anomalies and appear to be incompatible with long-term survival. Specifically, the skull in types 2 and 3 presents with the kleeblattschädel anomaly (cloverleaf skull) with severe shortening of the anterior skull base. Unlike type 2, type 3 Pfeiffer syndrome has anomalies of the gut, including prune belly and bowel malformations. Because types 2 and 3 are rarely encountered clinically because of early demise, Pfeiffer syndrome type 1 will be described in this section.

Speech Disorders: Articulation is impaired secondary to a Class III malocclusion caused by maxillary hypoplasia. The tongue tends to articulate in the mandibular arch with limited maxillary contact. All anterior sounds are distorted or substitutions made. These errors are obligatory and are related to the severity of the malocclusion. Anterior skeletal open-bite is common and results in lingual protrusion. Speech onset is delayed in a small percentage of cases secondary to neurologic complications such as hydrocephalus.

339

Feeding Disorders: Early feeding is often impaired secondary to airway compromise. Airway obstruction has multiple sources, including choanal atresia or stenosis, pharyngeal obstruction secondary to maxillary hypoplasia and the palate hanging deeply into the oropharynx, and in some cases, rigidity of the trachea caused by a solid cartilaginous tube rather than the normal ringlike structure.

Hearing Disorders: Conductive hearing loss is common, often reaching the moderate to severe range. Ossicular fusions have been found.

Voice Disorders: Hoarse voice is common, especially in cases with tracheal anomalies.

Resonance Disorders: Hyponasality is common secondary to choanal stenosis or atresia, and also because of maxillary hypoplasia that decreases the total volume of the nasopharyngeal airway. Oral resonance may also be impaired, with a muffled resonance caused by reduced maxillary volume and a reduction in oral cavity size.

Language Disorders: Language development is typically normal except in the small percentage of cases with neurological complications.

Other Clinical Features:

> **Craniofacial:** craniosynostosis of multiple sutures; acrocephaly; increased intracranial pressure; maxillary hypoplasia; shallow orbits; hypertelorism; downslanting palpebral fissures; choanal stenosis or atresia; soft tissue hypertrophy of the palatal shelves (pseudocleft); exophthalmos; Class III malocclusion;

> **Limbs:** broad thumbs and halluces; radially deviated thumbs; mild soft tissue syndactyly; brachydactyly; occasional polysyndactyly of the thumbs or halluces;

> **Central nervous system:** occasional hydrocephalus; occasional Arnold-Chiari anomaly.

Natural History: At birth, many babies with Pfeiffer syndrome have relatively normal facial appearance. Anthropometric measurement may yield evidence of hypertelorism. The anterior fontanel is often patent and remains that way through the first year of life. However, maxillary hypoplasia and acrocephaly become evident with growth. Increased intracranial pressure may also develop. With normal mandibular growth throughout childhood and maxillary hypoplasia, relative prognathism becomes evident before school age.

Treatment Prognosis: Craniofacial reconstruction can prevent the increase in intracranial pressure from becoming severe. Choanal stenosis or atresia cannot be permanently resolved with surgery because ossification of the craniofacial skeleton is progressive and continues throughout life. Airway obstruction may be life-threatening in many cases and tracheotomy is often necessary. Craniofacial reconstruction may be performed for the midfacial hypoplasia.

Differential Diagnosis: The craniofacial anomalies in Pfeiffer syndrome are similar to those seen in **Crouzon syndrome, Jackson-Weiss syndrome,** and **Apert syndrome.** The syndromes can be differentiated based on the limb anomalies. **Sathre-Chotzen syndrome** has similar soft tissue syndactyly of the hands, but the craniofacial anomalies are different than those found in Pfeiffer syndrome.

P

Pontobulbar Palsy With Sensorineural Hearing Loss

Also Known As: Brown-Vialetto-van Laere syndrome; progressive bulbar palsy with perceptive deafness

This syndrome of degenerative neurological complications is important to identify early because management of feeding disorders can be beneficial for avoiding potentially fatal complications of aspiration. Essentially all of the earliest manifestations of the disorder are communicative in nature, and audiologists and speech-language pathologists may often be the first professionals to come in contact with affected individuals.

Major System(s) Affected: Auditory; central nervous system.

Etiology: Autosomal recessive inheritance, autosomal dominant inheritance, and X-linked inheritance have all been hypothesized based on pedigree analysis of a number of families with multiple affected individuals. It is unclear if this represents etiologic heterogeneity versus a number of close phenocopies caused by different genes.

Speech Disorders: Speech onset and early development is normal. After the onset of the disease, weak oral consonant production follows. The tongue develops fasciculations followed by dysarthria.

Feeding Disorders: Dysphagia with aspiration and true bulbar-based disorders of swallowing eventually develop as the disease progresses. Diminished pharyngeal and laryngeal sensation and vocal cord paralysis are common in the end-stages of the disorder.

Hearing Disorders: In most cases, the first clinical expression of the syndrome is sensorineural hearing loss. Hearing loss usually appears in childhood in the primary school years, although some cases have demonstrated an early onset and others have not had clinical manifestations until late teen years.

Voice Disorders: Initially, voice is normal. After the onset of the disorder, voice is initially hoarse, followed by breathiness, and eventually dysphonia or aphonia related to vocal fold paresis occurs.

Resonance Disorders: An early manifestation of the disorder is the onset of hypernasal speech and nasal air emission.

Language Disorders: Language development is normal.

Other Clinical Features:

> **Auditory:** sensorineural hearing loss with occasionally very rapid progression;
>
> **Central nervous system:** lower cranial nerve palsies; lower motor neuron dysfunction; hypoactive reflexes; muscle wasting.

Natural History: The first noticeable symptom is usually hearing loss, although in some cases, upper eyelid ptosis may appear earlier. Hearing loss is followed by speech and resonance disorders, and then swallowing and respiratory complications. The disorder may have either very rapid or slow progression. In cases with rapid progression, early demise may occur secondary to respiratory complications, including diaphragmatic paresis, aspiration, and pulmonary insufficiency.

Treatment Prognosis: In cases with milder progression, alternative strategies for feeding may be very helpful in avoiding dangerous complications of bulbar palsy. Hypernasality will respond to prosthetic management, specifically obturation. Surgery is contraindicated because the disease is progressive.

Differential Diagnosis: There are a number of other rare disorders with similar progressive symptoms, including Fazio-Londe disease.

Popliteal Pterygium Syndrome

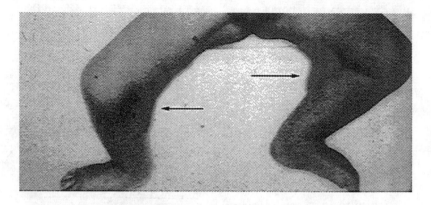

Arrows point to webbing of the popliteal space in popliteal pterygium syndrome.

Also Known As: Popliteal web syndrome; facio-genito-popliteal syndrome

Popliteal pterygium syndrome is one of a small number of disorders that display anomalies of the lower lip, specifically lower lip pits, in association with cleft palate or cleft lip and palate. It is also one of the syndromes that has mixing of cleft type within the same pedigree so that some individuals may have cleft lip and palate while others have cleft palate without cleft lip.

Major System(s) Affected: Craniofacial; limbs; genitals.

Etiology: Autosomal dominant inheritance. The gene has not been mapped or identified.

Speech Disorders: Articulation is often impaired by ankyloglossia and also by cleft anomalies of the maxillary alveolus and maxillary hypoplasia. The pits of the lower lip can result in an uneven vermilion line that can also result in articulatory distortions. There may also be compensatory articulation disorders secondary to cleft palate and velopharyngeal insufficiency.

Feeding Disorders: Infant feeding may be complicated by cleft anomalies, but is otherwise normal.

Hearing Disorders: Conductive hearing loss is common secondary to middle ear effusion.

Voice Disorders: Hoarse voice has been observed in some cases.

Resonance Disorders: Hypernasality secondary to cleft palate and velopharyngeal insufficiency is common.

Language Disorders: Language development is normal in most cases.

Other Clinical Features:

Craniofacial: cleft palate; cleft lip and palate; ankyloglossia; filiform adhesions of the eyelids; lower lip pits;

Limbs: popliteal pterygia; syndactyly of the fingers and toes; abnormal skin folds over the fingernails;

Genitals: hypoplastic labia and vagina; hypoplastic uterus; bifid scrotum; cryptorchidism.

Natural History: The popliteal webs and other anomalies are present at birth and with growth of the limbs cause progressive restriction of extension of the legs. Maxillary hypoplasia develops with age.

Treatment Prognosis: The popliteal webs are difficult to treat surgically because of abnormal nerves and blood vessels that run through the web spaces. Physical therapy and stretching may be of some limited value. Surgical correction of the other structural anomalies is indicated including removal of the lower lip pits.

Differential Diagnosis: Lower lip pits and clefts are found in **van der Woude syndrome,** but without the popliteal webbing.

Prader-Willi Syndrome

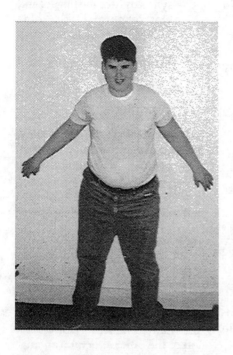

Prader-Willi syndrome.

Also Known As:

Prader-Willi syndrome is a relatively common contiguous gene syndrome that, along with **Angelman syndrome**, shows a pattern of inheritance known as imprinting. As does **Angelman syndrome**, Prader-Willi maps to 15q11. In many cases, the disorder is caused by deletion of 15q11.2-q12 from the paternal chromosome, or by maternal uniparental disomy. In other words, absence of the paternal 15q11 region results in Prader-Willi, but absence of the maternal 15q11 causes **Angelman syndrome.** Phenotypically, Prader-Willi and **Angelman syndromes** have few, if any similarities. One of the hallmarks of Prader-Willi syndrome is the obesity and constant voracious appetite displayed in childhood.

Major System(s) Affected:
Growth; central nervous system; craniofacial; ocular; genitourinary; musculoskeletal; integument.

Etiology: Absence of paternal 15q11 chromosome region that can occur as a result of deletion from the paternal chromosome 15, or maternal uniparental disomy of chromosome 15.

Speech Disorders: Misarticulations are common, particularly weak oral contacts, omissions of final sounds, and distortions, primarily related to hypotonia and, in some cases, secondary to velopharyngeal insufficiency.

Feeding Disorders: In the neonatal period, severe hypotonia leads to poor suck, poor feeding, and airway obstruction that further interferes with feeding. Although failure-to-thrive is a common feature in infancy, in toddler years, children begin to become obese even though they do not consume an enormous amount of calories. Children with Prader-Willi syndrome often become hyperphagic, usually engaging in binge eating. Their attempts to get food are often very persistent, requiring parents to engage in strategies to prevent them from reaching food.

Hearing Disorders: Hearing is normal in Prader-Willi syndrome.

Voice Disorders: Voice is often initially weak in infancy, but eventually reaches normal strength.

Resonance Disorders: Hypernasality in the absence of cleft palate is a frequent finding in childhood and is secondary to hypotonia.

Language Disorders: Language development is essentially always delayed, but the initial signs of cognitive impairment and language delay appear worse than they really are because the hypotonia is so severe. Following initial delay, there is substantial catch-up in terms of language and intellectual development.

Other Clinical Features:

Growth: short stature; obesity;

Central nervous system: severe hypotonia; cognitive impairment; maladaptive behaviors; sleep disturbance; hyporeflexia; self-destructive

P

behavior; high tolerance for pain;

Craniofacial: bitemporal narrowing; thin upper lip; upslanting almond-shaped eyes;

Ocular: strabismus; myopia;

Genitourinary: hypogonadism; cryptorchidism; hypoplastic labia; amenorrhea;

Musculoskeletal: small hands and feet; scoliosis; kyphosis; osteopenia;

Integument: hypopigmentation;

Other: decreased fetal movements; poor control of body temperature.

Natural History: The lack of vigorous fetal movments is often the first clinical sign of Prader-Willi syndrome. At birth, hypotonia is very severe and makes the prognosis for psychomotor development seem poor in infancy. Failure-to-thrive in infancy is very common, but is replaced in childhood by hyperphagia and obesity. Expressive language is particularly delayed, but eventually improves. Children with Prader-Willi have been de-scribed as affectionate, happy, and good-natured. However, behavior often becomes difficult with temper tantrums, bouts of rage, and stubborn behavior. Hypernasality is a common finding in childhood, but is not related to cleft palate or submucous cleft palate. Rather, hypotonia results in a general lack of movement of the velopharyngeal mechanism. With age, muscle tone improves dramatically, and hypernasality typically resolves spontaneously.

Treatment Prognosis: With proper behavioral management, hyperphagia can be controlled and obesity prevented. Hypogonadism responds well to testosterone treatment in males. Response to speech therapy, physical therapy, and occupational therapy can be excellent. Cognitive impairment is constant, but is typically in the mild to moderate range, some cases having borderline normal intellect.

Differential Diagnosis: Other syndromes with obesity and hypotonia as clinical features include the **Bardet-Biedl syndromes** and **Laurence-Moon syndrome.** Hypotonia with early overgrowth is seen in **Beckwith-Wiedemann syndrome.**

Proteus Syndrome

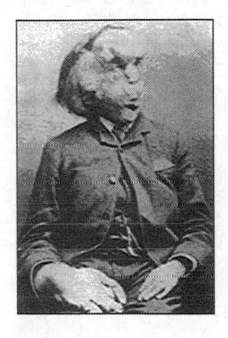

John Merrick (labeled the Elephant Man), *who has been determined to have had Proteus syndrome.*

Also Known As:

Proteus syndrome is best known because it is likely that the so-called *Elephant Man* popularized in a film by the same name had this disorder, although some people mistakenly believe he had neurofibromatosis. The syndrome is named *Proteus* because the Greek god Proteus had the ability to change shapes at will and individuals with Proteus syndrome have dramatic alterations in their physical phenotype over time because of the growth of multiple severe hamartomas.

Major System(s) Affected:

Craniofacial; integument; ocular; renal; central nervous system; skeletal.

Etiology: Unknown. All cases have been sporadic.

349

Speech Disorders: Speech may be impaired by either structural anomalies or neurogenic abnormalities. Overgrowth and disortion of the maxilla and mandible may make tongue movement and placement difficult, and may be exacerbated by the presence of oral tumors. Individuals with central nervous system impairment (probably less than half of affected individuals) are also likely to have dysarthria.

Feeding Disorders: Early feeding is not typically impaired because most affected individuals are normal at birth, but with continued growth of hamartomas, feeding may become impaired by a combination of airway problems and malocclusion. A soft diet occasionally becomes necessary if the overgrowth is severe.

Hearing Disorders: Hearing loss has not been documented or observed.

Voice Disorders: Voice may become hoarse in relation to distortion of laryngeal suspension caused by cervical spinal anomalies.

Resonance Disorders: Resonance may become hyponasal with progression of multiple tumors. Oral resonance often becomes muffled because of oral skeletal overgrowth and soft tissue overgrowth of the lips and cheeks.

Language Disorders: Language development is normal in most cases, but those with central nervous system impairment will have language delay and impairment.

Other Clinical Features:

Craniofacial: hyperostoses of the calvarium; skeletal overgrowth of the maxilla and mandible; macrocephaly;

Integument: multiple hamartomas; lymphangioma; lipomas; hamartomas of the soles of the feet; pigmentary anomalies;

Ocular: epibulbar growths;

Renal: renal anomalies;

Central nervous system: cognitive deficiency in approximately half of known cases; brain anomalies; compression of the spinal cord;

Skeletal: kyphoscoliosis.

Natural History: Most affected individuals appear normal at birth, but abnormal growth begins in early childhood in most cases. When severe, the progression of the disorder can threaten life if respiratory obstruction becomes severe.

Treatment Prognosis: Palliative treatment with specific tumor removals may prove useful for short-term gain, but long-term prognosis depends on the severity of expression.

Differential Diagnosis: Craniofacial and somatic asymmetry are common and when associated with facial hyperostoses, the disorder may initially resemble hemihypertrophy. However, the presence of tumors and hamartomas differentiates Proteus syndrome.

Pycnodysostosis

Also Known As: Pyknodysotosis

Pycnodysostosis is a syndrome of short stature that has osteosclerosis and tendency for the bones to fracture. It is a rare but easily recognized disorder. It has been suggested, and is probably true, that the French artist Toulouse-Lautrec had pycnodysostosis.

Major System(s) Affected: skeletal; growth; craniofacial; dental; limbs; hematologic; visceral; central nervous system.

Etiology: Autosomal recessive inheritance. The gene has been mapped to 1q21.

Speech Disorders: Articulation is often marked by distortions, particularly those caused by tongue protrusion related to hypodontia and anterior skeletal open-bite related to steep mandibular plane angle. Intelligibility, however, is typically good.

Feeding Disorders: Feeding is not typically impaired.

Hearing Disorders: Hearing is within normal limits in pycnodysostosis.

Voice Disorders: Voice is "tinny," thin, and high-pitched.

Resonance Disorders: Nasal resonance is normal, but oral resonance is often muffled because the pharynx is vertically short.

Language Disorders: Language is normal in most cases, but is impaired in the small percentage of cases with cognitive impairment.

Other Clinical Features:

> **Skeletal:** osteosclerosis; fragile bones with frequent fractures; spinal anomalies; hypoplastic clavicles; hip dislocation; short limbs;
>
> **Growth:** short stature;
>
> **Craniofacial:** brachycephaly; round face; widely patent cranial sutures; micrognathia; midface deficiency; steep mandibular plane angle;
>
> **Dental:** hypodontia; delayed dental eruption;
>
> **Limbs:** brachydactyly;
>
> **Hematologic:** anemia;

Visceral: hepatosplenomegaly;

Central nervous system: occasional cognitive impairpairment.

Natural History: The risk of fractures increases with age. The mandible, clavicle, and legs are particularly susceptible to fractures. The osteosclerosis is progressive. Late dental eruption and hypodontia add to the malocclusion that can impair speech.

Treatment Prognosis: The facial skeleton is disproportionate with malocclusion that may lead some clinicians to suggest reconstructive surgery. However, the bones are brittle and may shatter during orthognathic surgery. Dental implants would also be problematic. Even prosthetic dental restorations present a challenge if too many teeth are missing.

Differential Diagnosis: Persistently patent cranial sutures and clavicular hypoplasia are found in **cleidocranial dysplasia,** and the limb findings are also somewhat similar. However, the craniofacial features of pycnodysostosis are different, without the broad bifurcated forehead typical of **cleidocranial dysplasia.** Acroosteolysis has similar skeletal and facial findings.

P

Rapp-Hodgkin Syndrome

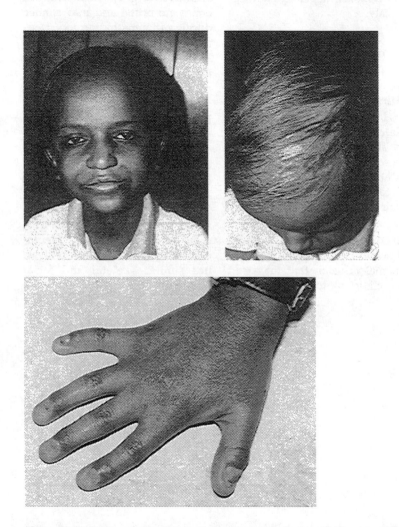

Rapp-Hodgkin syndrome: Note the sparse scalp hair and absence of the fingernails.

Also Known As: Hypohidrotic ectodermal dysplasia with cleft lip and cleft palate

Rapp-Hodgkin syndrome is one of the syndromes of clefting that can express mixing of cleft type within a single pedigree. Individuals with Rapp-Hodgkin can have cleft lip with cleft palate or cleft palate alone in association with the ectodermal dysplasia that represents the other major feature of the syndrome.

Major System(s) Affected: Integument; craniofacial, dental; genitals; ocular.

Etiology: Autosomal dominant inheritance. The gene has not been mapped or identified.

Speech Disorders: Articulation disorders include obligatory distortions and substitutions secondary to small or missing teeth. The cleft anomalies of the lip, dental alveolus, and palate may also result in compensatory articulation patterns.

Feeding Disorders: Early feeding may be complicated by the cleft, but no other infantile feeding difficulties occur. In later life, missing teeth may complicate chewing.

Hearing Disorders: Conductive hearing loss secondary to chronic otitis media is common and is related to the cleft anomaly.

Voice Disorders: Voice is hoarse because of hypohidrosis and drying of the vocal cords.

Resonance Disorders: Hypernasal resonance secondary to cleft palate and velopharyngeal insufficiency may occur.

Language Disorders: Language is normal. Cognitive impairment is not a feature of Rapp-Hodgkin syndrome.

Other Clinical Features:

Integument: anhidrotic/hypohidrotic ectodermal dysplasia; coarse, wiry, and sparse scalp hair; eventual alopecia; dysplastic nails;

Craniofacial: cleft palate with or without cleft lip; narrow nose;

Dental: hypodontia;

Genitals: hypospadias;

Ocular: tearing abnormalities.

Natural History: If no cleft is present, the anomalies associated with Rapp-Hodgkin dysplasia may be difficult to detect at birth because infants have no teeth and many have no hair. Infant nails also tend to be soft and very small. Unexplained fevers may not immediately be linked to hypohidrosis. Delayed or absent eruption of teeth and dysplastic hair and nails help to confirm the diagnosis.

Treatment Prognosis: All anomalies can be treated symptomatically and the prognosis is excellent. If any secondary teeth are present, prosthetic replacement is possible. Deficiency of alveolar bone may compromise the use of dental implants.

Differential Diagnosis: The syndrome has significant phenotypic overlap with **AEC syndrome** (Hay-Wells syndrome). The presence of filiform adhesions on the eyelids is consistent with AEC syndrome, but not Rapp-Hodgkin syndrome.

Robinow Syndrome

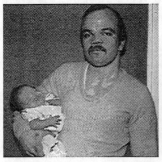 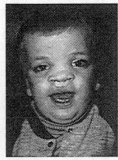 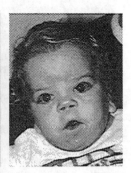

Robinow syndrome: Father and his two affected sons, one with cleft lip and palate, and the other with a submucous cleft palate, but no cleft lip.

Also Known As: Fetal face syndrome

Robinow syndrome is a relatively rare multiple anomaly disorder that has the combination of craniofacial, genital, skeletal, and growth anomalies, but it is probably underrecognized in cleft palate and craniofacial centers. Cleft palate with or without cleft lip is a common anomaly in the syndrome, and like **van der Woude syndrome, Rapp-Hodgkin syndrome, craniofrontonasal syndrome,** and **EEC syndrome,** among others, it is one of a group of syndromes that may express different cleft types (cleft palate alone and cleft palate with cleft lip) among first degree relatives. This type of mixing of cleft types only occurs in syndromes, and is not found in nonsyndromic clefting.

Major System(s) Affected: Craniofacial; growth; genitals; skeletal.

Etiology: Autosomal dominant inheritance has been confirmed, but many cases with autosomal recessive inheritance have also been reported. It is unclear if the dominant and recessive forms represent the same disorder or similar syndromes with different genetic etiologies. The gene(s) for the disorder have not been mapped or identified. Opportunities to observe dominant cases are probably reduced because of hypogenitalism in affected males.

Speech Disorders: Articulation impairment secondary to malocclusion is common with the errors being obligatory in nature. Compensatory articulation patterns related to cleft palate and velopharyngeal insufficiency may also occur.

Feeding Disorders: Feeding disorders have not been reported or observed.

Hearing Disorders: Conductive hearing loss secondary to cleft palate and chronic middle ear effusion may occur.

Voice Disorders: Voice is typically normal in Robinow syndrome.

Resonance Disorders: Hypernasality may occur secondary to cleft palate and velopharyngeal insufficiency. A cul-de-sac resonance may also occur because of a small nose anteriorly.

Language Disorders: Language and intellect are normal in almost all cases, but several instances of mental retardation have been reported. It is unclear if this is a firm component of the syndrome.

Other Clinical Features:

Craniofacial: macrocephaly; hypertelorism; wide palpebral fissures; short nose; depressed nasal root; frontal bossing; thickened calvarium; osteosclerosis; retrognathia; platybasia; cleft palate with or without cleft lip;

Growth: short stature;

Genitals: micropenis; hypoplastic clitoris and labia majora; cryptorchidism; ambiguous genitalia on occasion;

Skeletal: vertebral anomalies; osteochondrodysplasia;

Limbs: shortening of the forearms; brachydactyly; broad thumbs with occasional bifurcation of the distal phalanx.

Natural History: Facial appearance at birth is often indistinguishable from normal, but the craniofacial manifestations of the syndrome become more obvious with growth. The shortening of the forearms is also difficult to detect initially. The cranium appears large, especially in relation to the face, but with age, there is marked thickening of the calvarium. Hypoplasia of the genitals is the one finding that is more obvious at birth.

Treatment Prognosis: The prognosis is generally excellent.

Differential Diagnosis: Although the short stature is not as severe, the facial appearance and disproportion of the limbs is similar to that seen in **achondroplasia.**

R

Rubinstein-Taybi Syndrome

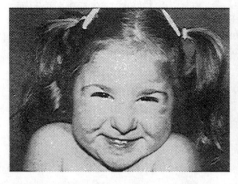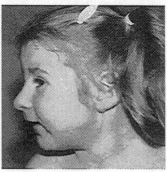

Rubinstein-Taybi syndrome.

Also Known As: Rubinstein syndrome; broad thumb-hallux syndrome

Rubinstein-Taybi syndrome is a relatively common syndrome of mental retardation among individuals who are institutionalized. The population frequency is low, perhaps 1: 300,000. The combination of distinctive craniofacial, developmental, heart, and limb anomalies is easily recognized.

Major System(s) Affected: Central nervous system; craniofacial; growth; limbs; cardiac; integument; ocular; musculoskeletal; gastrointestinal; genitourinary.

Etiology: Autosomal dominant inheritance. The gene has been mapped to 16p13.3 and the gene has been labeled CBP for CREB Binding Protein and mutations of this gene, including deletions, have been identified. The CBP gene acts to bind two proteins together and this binding process eventually activates other genes. Mutations in CBP prevent the binding, and thus the activation, of other genes.

Speech Disorders: A high percentage of individuals with Rubinstein-Taybi syndrome do not develop speech. Those who do develop speech usually display severe impairment of articulation, rhythm, and rate, often with significant dysarthria. Children are often labeled as dyspraxic. Speech is often unintelligible.

Feeding Disorders: Early failure-to-thrive is common and is precipitated by hypotonia, congenital heart anomalies, micrognathia, laryngomalacia, and airway obstruction. Chronic constipation also contributes to abdominal discomfort that decreases desire to feed.

Hearing Disorders: Conductive hearing loss is found in nearly a quarter of individuals with Rubinstein-Taybi syndrome.

Voice Disorders: Hoarseness and high pitch have been observed in many cases.

Resonance Disorders: Hypernasal resonance has been observed as a component of dysarthric speech and related to hypotonia. However, even when present, hypernasality has not been a major contributor to unintelligibility as has the speech production disorder.

Language Disorders: Language impairment is a constant, and expressive language is always more severely impaired than receptive language. Many individuals with Rubinstein-Taybi syndrome have good language comprehension but have essentially no functional speech.

Other Clinical Features:

Central nervous system: mental retardation, typically moderate, with the majority of IQs below 50; seizures; hyperactive deep tendon reflexes; hypoplasia or absence of the corpus callosum; hypotonia; psychiatric illness;

Craniofacial: microcephaly; large anterior fontanelle; mild hypertelorism; downslanting eyes; micrognathia; mild facial asymmetry; beak-shaped nose; downslanting oral commissures; long eyelashes;

Growth: short stature;

Limbs: broad thumbs and halluces; hyperextensible joints; radially deviated thumbs; broad distal phalanges on all digits;

Cardiac: venticular and atrial septal defects; patent ductus arteriosus; coarctation of the aorta; conduction abnormalities; pulmonary stenosis; mitral valve insufficiency; cardiomyopathy; cor pulmonale;

Integument: hirsutism; capillary hemangiomas; supernumerary nipples; keloid formation;

Ocular: strabismus; nasolacrimal duct obstruction; ptosis; ocular coloboma; cataracts; glaucoma;

Musculoskeletal: spina bifida occulta; scoliosis; kyphosis; frequent fractures; abnormal femoral epiphyses; short sternum;

Gastrointestinal: constipation, aganglionic megacolon;

Genitourinary: renal hypoplasia/aplasia; cryptorchidism.

Natural History: The facial manifestations of Rubinstein-Taybi syndrome are not always obvious at birth or in infancy, and broadening of the thumbs and halluces is difficult to appreciate when the hands and feet are very small. Therefore, many cases of Rubinstein-Taybi syndrome are diagnosed relatively late in life, often during childhood or at school age. One of the earliest presentations if heart anomalies are

not present is failure-to-thrive and chronic constipation, followed by developmental delay. The onset of speech is usually severely delayed. In many individuals with Rubinstein-Taybi syndrome who do develop speech, the onset of first words may not occur until 3 or 4 years of age. In many cases, speech consists of a small sample of single words. In those with more speech development, speech is often unintelligible. As adolescence approaches, maladaptive behaviors become more common and psychiatric illness involving mood and temperament become evident in many cases.

Treatment Prognosis: The prognosis for normal speech development is typically poor. In many cases, because receptive language is more intact, the potential for expressive language might appear good. However, if the onset of significant speech does not occur by school age, the prognosis for considerable speech development is typically poor.

Differential Diagnosis: Broad thumbs and halluces, as well as beaked nose and hypertelorism, are common findings in **Pfeiffer syndrome.** However, the presence of heart anomalies would negate the diagnosis of Pfeiffer. Because of the unusual facial appearance in Rubinstein-Taybi syndrome, the diagnosis of **de Lange syndrome** has been made incorrectly in some cases. Coarctation of the aorta, ASD, VSD, developmental delay, severe speech delay, psychiatric illness, and unusual facial appearance are also found in **velo-cardio-facial syndrome,** but there is little similarity in the facial phenotype with advancing age.

Saethre-Chotzen Syndrome

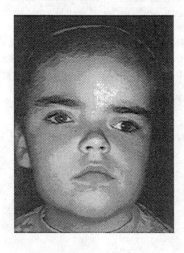

Saethre-Chotzen syndrome: Note orbital and facial asymmetry.

Also Known As: Acrocephalo-syndactyly, type III

Sathre-Chotzen syndrome is one of the least recognized and diagnosed syndromes of craniosynostosis. There is little resemblance between Saethre-Chotzen and **Crouzon, Apert,** or **Pfeiffer syndromes** even though Saethre-Chotzen syndrome has been labeled as one of the acro-cephalosyndactyly disorders.

Major System(s) Affected: Craniofacial; limbs; ocular; cardiac; central nervous system.

Etiology: Autosomal dominant inheritance. The gene has been mapped to 7p21 and has been iden-tified as the TWIST transcription factor gene.

Speech Disorders: In the small percentage of cases with cognitive impairment, there may be delayed onset of speech development. Speech production is otherwise typically normal.

Feeding Disorders: Feeding disorders have not been reported or observed.

Hearing Disorders: Conductive hearing loss is relatively common, but not a constant finding. In some cases, the hearing loss is unilateral and is typically mild to moderate.

Voice Disorders: Voice production is normal.

Resonance Disorders: Nasal resonance disorders of both types have been observed, including hypernasality secondary to cleft palate and velopharyngeal insufficiency and hyponasality secondary to reduced diameter of the nasopharynx.

Language Disorders: Language is impaired in a small percentage of cases, specifically those that have cognitive impairment.

Other Clinical Features:

Craniofacial: craniosynostosis; craniofacial asymmetry; brachycephaly; acrocephaly; cleft palate;

Limbs: lack of extension at elbows and knees; mild soft tissue syndactyly;

Ocular: strabismus;

Cardiac: occasional congenital heart anomalies;

Central nervous system: occasional cognitive impairment.

Natural History: In many instances, the craniosynostosis is evident at birth and may appear to be severe, but cranial growth and shape often improves with age. Development is typically normal.

Treatment Prognosis: The prognosis is typically good and reconstructive surgery may be effective in treating craniofacial and limb anomalies.

Differential Diagnosis: Saethre-Chotzen syndrome is not typically misdiagnosed as one of the other syndromes of craniosynostosis, but the clinical findings are more typically attributed to simple isolated craniosynostosis or plagiocephaly.

Sanfilippo Syndrome

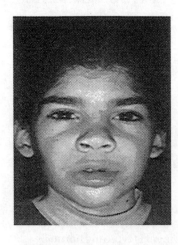

Coarse facial appearance in Sanfilippo syndrome.

Also Known As: Mucopolysaccharidosis type III, with subtypes Mucopolysaccharidosis type IIIA, IIIB, IIIC, and IIID, or as Sanfilippo A, B, C, or D. The difference between the four subtypes is the gene causing the phenotype and the specific enzyme deficiency

Sanfilippo syndrome is another of the lysosomal storage diseases known as the mucopolysaccharidoses. Several variants of Sanfilippo syndrome have been delineated, each caused by a different gene, but with similar phenotypes. Some estimates for the birth frequency of Sanfilippo syndrome are as high as 1:24,000.

Major System(s) Affected: Growth; craniofacial; central nervous system; musculoskeletal; integument; hepatic.

Etiology: All four subtypes are autosomal recessive disorders. The gene for Sanfilippo A causes a deficiency of heparan N-sulfatase and has been mapped to 17q25.3. The gene for Sanfilippo B has been mapped to 17q21, Sanfilippo C to chromosome 14, and Sanfilippo D to 12q14.

Speech Disorders: Early speech milestones are typically normal, but in early childhood, developmental delay becomes apparent. Any speech that is attained in childhood is eventually lost.

Feeding Disorders: Early feeding is normal, but with advancing expression of the disorder, there is chronic airway difficulty and deteriorating neurologic function that results in difficulty feeding. Eventual loss of bulbar function makes normal oral feeding impossible.

Hearing Disorders: Conductive hearing loss secondary to chronic and severe middle ear effusion is common and progressive. Onset is typically at about school age.

Voice Disorders: Voice becomes hoarse with the progression of the disorder. There may be a behavioral component because children become aggressive and many have temper tantrums with screaming.

Resonance Disorders: Resonance eventually becomes hyponasal as chronic mucus fills the nasal cavity and mucous membranes become boggy. There is eventual loss of bulbar function.

Language Disorders: Early language milestones are normal, but delay becomes evident in childhood and deterioration follows.

Other Clinical Features:

Growth: short stature, typically mild;

Craniofacial: thick calvarial bones; mildly coarse face; macrocephaly;

Central nervous system: eventual mental retardation with progressive deterioration; hyperactivity; aggressiveness; ADD/ADHD; frequent and severe temper tantrums; destructive behavior;

Musculoskeletal: anomalous vertebrae; stiffening of the joints;

Integument: hirsutism;

Hepatic: mild liver enlargement.

Natural History: The onset of the disorder is typically apparent early in the toddler stage as developmental milestones begin to lag behind. An early sign is overactive and aggressive behavior, which is usually apparent before any significant coarsening of the facies. There is often severe sleep disturbance, including both restlessness and eventually obstructive sleep apnea. Eventually, motor control becomes severely impaired. There is progressive ataxia, dementia, seizures, tremors, and eventual bulbar dysfunction that can prevent normal feeding. Most affected individuals do not survive beyond 20 years of age.

Treatment Prognosis: Extremely poor.

Differential Diagnosis: The phenotype and progressive nature of the disorder is similar to other lysosomal storage diseases and metabolic disorders. There are definitive molecular tests that can confirm the diagnosis of Sanfilippo syndrome (for all types).

Seitelberger Syndrome

Also Known As: Infantile neuroaxonal dystrophy; Seitelberger disease

Seitelberger syndrome is a degenerative neurological disorder of infancy that is probably one of the most common disorders of its type. The disorder has a rapid progressive course that ultimately results in the child's demise, with feeding, speech, and hearing disorders all common manifestations of the syndrome.

Major System(s) Affected: Central nervous system; ocular; endocrine; circulation.

Etiology: Autosomal recessive inheritance. The gene has not been mapped or identified.

Speech Disorders: Initial speech milestones are normal, typically developing to approximately 2 years of age. Development then stagnates, and eventually all acquired motor activities deteriorate and are lost. Speech is lost entirely, sometimes within months of onset of the disorder.

Feeding Disorders: Initially, feeding is normal, but the initial onset of the disorder is marked by hypotonia followed by hyperactive reflexes, poor head control, abnormal posturing, and finally total loss of motor control, including gastrointestinal and esophageal function.

Hearing Disorders: Toward the end of the progression of the syndrome, sensorineural hearing loss occurs. The hearing loss is difficult to detect because it is accompanied by severe neurologic degeneration and dementia.

Voice Disorders: Initially, voice is normal, but at the onset of the degenerative process, hoarseness and breathiness are common.

Resonance Disorders: Initially resonance is normal. With the onset of neurological degeneration, hypernasality is likely to occur and become progressively more severe.

Language Disorders: Initially, language development is normal. Following the onset of the disorder, language stagnates and then degenerates until all useful language function is lost.

Other Clinical Features:

Central nervous system: CNS degeneration; brain swelling; axonal degeneration; seizures; hypotonia; abnormal reflexes;

Ocular: nystagmus; absence of tearing;

Endocrine: hypothyroidism; diabetes insipidus; lack of control of autonomic function, including temperature regulation;

Circulation: distal gangrene.

Natural History: Early development is normal, including all psychomotor milestones. The onset of observable symptoms is at approximately 2 years in many cases, but earlier symptoms have been observed. Within months of onset, significant neurological degeneration becomes evident with total loss of psychomotor milestones eventually occurring. Death occurs in nearly all cases within a decade of the onset of the initial findings.

Treatment Prognosis: The progression of the disorder cannot be halted and palliative treatment is not available.

Differential Diagnosis: The onset of a degenerative process in infancy or toddler years occurs in many of the lysosomal storage disorders, such as **Hurler syndrome** and **Hunter syndrome.** However, these disorders are characterized by significant progression of abnormal physical abnormalities related to intracellular storage of glycosaminoglycans.

Setleis Syndrome

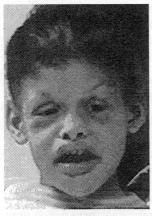 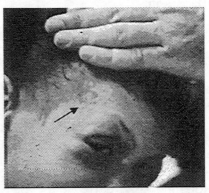

Loose facial skin and temporal "forceps marks" (arrow) in Setleis syndrome.

Also Known As: Facial ectodermal dysplasia; bitemporal forceps marks syndrome; focal facial dermal dysplasia, type II. The majority of early cases were from Puerto Rico, but cases from other racial and ethnic groups have subsequently been identified.

Setleis syndrome is a rare but very distinctive syndrome involving multiple anomalies of the face primarily focused on the skin. Although individuals with Setleis syndrome are cognitively normal, their appearance is so stigmatizing that it may result in social isolation and its potential consequences.

Major System(s) Affected: Integument; craniofacial; gastrointestinal.

Etiology: Presumed to be autosomal recessive because of multiple affected siblings from normal parents, and several isolated cases from consanguineous parents.

Speech Disorders: Articulation has been impaired related to distor-

S

tions of bilabial and labiodental sounds secondary to loose, redundant facial skin.

Feeding Disorders: Feeding is normal.

Hearing Disorders: Hearing loss has not been observed.

Voice Disorders: Voice production is normal.

Resonance Disorders: Resonance balance is normal.

Language Disorders: Language development has been delayed in a single case seen by the author, but has otherwise been noted as normal.

Other Clinical Features:

Integument: Loose, wrinkled facial skin resulting in an aged appearance; deep marks in the temporal area that look like forceps marks; hypermobility of the facial skin; multiple rows of eyelashes;

Craniofacial: puffy upper eyelids; depressed nasal root; upslanting eyebrows; bulbous nasal tip;

Gastrointestinal: imperforate anus.

Natural History: The skin anomalies and unusual facial appearance are present at birth. The abnormality becomes more severe with age.

Treatment Prognosis: There is not a significant experience with surgical management of the facial disorder, but surgical reconstruction is certainly indicated to tighten the facial skin and eliminate the redundancy.

Differential Diagnosis: Another similar disorder, Brauer syndrome, has been regarded by some clinicians to be the same disorder as Setleis syndrome, but this hypothesis has not been confirmed. Otherwise, the clinical manifestations of Setleis syndrome are essentially unique.

SHORT Syndrome

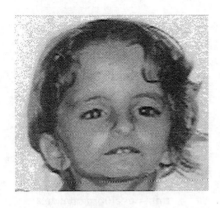

SHORT syndrome.

Also Known As: Short stature, lipoatrophy, and Rieger anomaly

The appelation of SHORT syndrome is another attempt to match an acronym to one of the major findings associated with the disorder, as in **LEOPARD syndrome.** Short stature is one of the major findings in this multiple anomaly disorder, along with a distinctive facial appearance and Rieger anomaly, an eye abnormality involving maldevelopment of the anterior chamber of the eye resulting in abnormal appearance of the iris and pupil.

Major System(s) Affected: Growth; craniofacial; ocular; musculoskeletal; dental; central nervous system.

Etiology: Autosomal recessive inheritance. The gene has not been mapped or identified.

Speech Disorders: Speech onset is delayed, usually more significantly than the degree of developmental delay would suggest. Articulation impairment is also common, related to delayed dental eruption and micrognathia.

Feeding Disorders: Feeding disorders have not been reported or observed.

Hearing Disorders: Sensorineural hearing loss is an occasional manifestation of the disorder.

Voice Disorders: Voice is typically high-pitched.

Resonance Disorders: Abnormal resonance characteristics have not been observed or reported.

Language Disorders: Language delay is common, with expressive language impairment more impaired than receptive. The specific role of hearing impairment in relation to the language delay has not been determined, but because language impairment is a more common finding than hearing loss, it is likely that the language impairment is a primary anomaly associated with the syndrome.

Other Clinical Features:

Growth: short stature; low birth weight; lipoatrophy;

Craniofacial: absence of facial fat; triangular facial shape; deep-set eyes; micrognathia; downturned oral commissures;

Ocular: Rieger anomaly; anomalies of the iris and cornea; neonatal glaucoma;

Musculoskeletal: hyperextensible joints; congenital hip dislocation; inguinal hernia; delayed bone age;

Dental: delayed dental eruption;

Central nervous system: mild developmental delay.

Natural History: Mild developmental delay may be related to mild hypotonia and musculoskeletal weakness, but the severity of expressive language impairment makes the degree of psychomotor impairment look worse initially. With growth and age, the severity of lipoatrophy makes the children look increasingly dysmorphic, often giving them a prematurely aged appearance. Some cases have experienced chronic respiratory illness. Others have developed diabetes mellitus.

Treatment Prognosis: The prognosis is essentially good and symptomatic and palliative treatments should be effective.

Differential Diagnosis: The facies is similar to that seen in Granddad syndrome, and has some similarities to **Bloom syndrome,** Cockayne syndrome, and progeria because of the prematurely aged appearance.

Shprintzen-Goldberg Syndrome

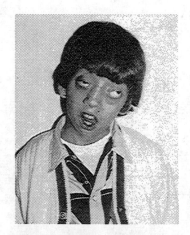

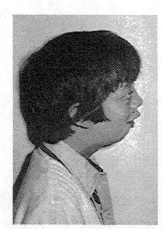

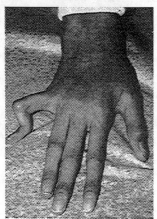

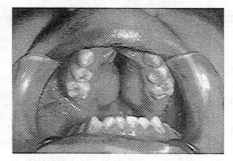

Exorbitism, micrognathia, cervical spine anomalies (top row), arachnodactyly, and pseudocleft of the hard palate in Shprintzen-Goldberg syndrome.

Also Known As: Shprintzen-Goldberg craniosynostosis syndrome; Marfanoid craniosynostosis syndrome; craniosynostosis with arachnodactyly and abdominal hernias.

Shprintzen-Goldberg syndrome is a rare and unusual disorder with typically severe craniofacial manifestations in association with multiple connective tissue disorders and joint abnormalities. Cognitive impairment is a common finding, as is respiratory obstruction. Over a dozen cases have been described in the scientific literature, but the syndrome is clearly underdiagnosed and may be confused with Marfan syndrome or Crouzon syndrome in some cases.

Major System(s) Affected: Craniofacial; central nervous system; musculoskeletal; cardiovascular.

Etiology: Unknown. A single report described a mutation in the same fibrillin gene that causes Marfan syndrome, but mutations in fibrillin have not been found in all other patients previously identified and it is likely that the case described with a fibrillin mutation does not have the syndrome.

Speech Disorders: Severely delayed onset in speech in many, but not all, cases. Articulation is often very impaired because of severe restriction of oral cavity size and because of severe hypotonia. There is marked soft tissue hypertrophy of the lateral palatal shelves secondary to a chronic mouth-open posture and hypotonia with lack of tongue movement in the maxillary arch. Anterior skeletal open-bite is essentially constant, even in early childhood causing lingual protrusion disorders. Dysarthria is common.

Feeding Disorders: Early feeding is difficult secondary to chronic upper airway obstruction related to an extremely short anterior cranial base. Later in life, chewing large pieces of food is difficult because of severe malocclusion and anterior skeletal open-bite.

Hearing Disorders: Hearing abnormalities have not been reported or observed.

Voice Disorders: Hoarse voice has been observed in several cases.

Resonance Disorders: Hyponasality secondary to nasal airway obstruction is common.

Language Disorders: Language is often severely delayed and impaired.

Other Clinical Features:

Craniofacial: craniosynostosis of multiple sutures; dolicocephaly; low-set posteriorly rotated ears; soft pliable external ears; exophthalmos; maxillary and mandibular hypoplasia; soft tissue hypertrophy of the palatal shelved with "pseudocleft"; short anterior skull base; choanal atresia or stenosis;

Central nervous system: cognitive impairment;

Limbs: arachnodactyly; camptodactyly;

Musculoskeletal: multiple abdominal hernias; scoliosis; kyphosis; atlanto-occipital instability; cervical spine anomalies; pectus excavatum or carinatum; limited joint mobility; marfanoid habitus;

Cardiovascular: dilitation of the aortic root; aortic dissection;

Ocular: strabismus.

Natural History: Early development is typically severely delayed. Ambulation is often difficult because of the combined effects of hypotonia and joint limitations. Cervical spine anomalies may also impinge on the spinal cord and cause damage resulting in neurological sequelae. Respiratory obstruction is often noted in the neonatal period and may become progressively worse with age because of the advancing effects of failure for the anterior skull base to grow. The facial abnormalities become progressively worse over time. Early death has been observed in a number of cases secondary to respiratory compromise or aortic dissection. Although speech is severely delayed and may be dysarthric, speech does typically develop.

Treatment Prognosis: Treatment prognosis has been poor in cases followed to date because of progressive worsening of the respiratory compromise and combined effects of musculoskeletal (especially spinal) and neurological abnormalities. However, speech therapy is clearly indicated, and in surviving patients, skeletal surgery to resolve craniofacial anomalies is certainly indicated.

Differential Diagnosis: Marfan syndrome has similar somatic effects, but the craniofacial manifestations are different. Several cases have been incorrectly identified as Crouzon syndrome because of the craniosynostosis and exophthalmos. However, the limb anomalies in Shprintzen-Goldberg syndrome are unique in syndromes of craniosynostosis.

Smith-Lemli-Opitz Syndrome

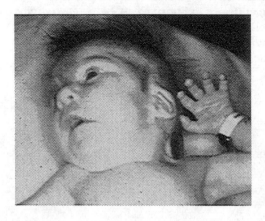

Smith-Lemli-Opitz syndrome: Note micrognathia, short nose with anteverted nostrils, and square, high forehead.

Also Known As: Smith-Lemli-Opitz, type I; RSH syndrome

Smith-Lemli-Opitz syndrome (SLO) was labeled RSH syndrome by John Opitz, using the initials of the names of the first three families in whom the diagnosis was made. The disorder's cardinal features include mental retardation, genital anomalies, and growth deficiency with a high frequency of neonatal and infant death. Some clinicians have suggested that there are two forms of SLO, type I (typical manifestations) and type II (more severe manifestations), but it is likely that both of these subtypes represent variable expression of the same disorder. However, many patients do survive with varying degrees of mental retardation and typically severe language and speech impairment. The syndrome has a birth frequency of approximately 1:20,000.

Major System(s) Affected: Central nervous system; growth; craniofacial; genitourinary; cardiopulmonary; gastrointestinal; limbs; metabolic.

Etiology: Autosomal recessive inheritance. The gene has been mapped to 11q12-q13 and has been identified as DHCR7, dehydrocholesterol reductase 7.

Speech Disorders: A substantial percentage of individuals with SLO do not develop functional speech, and many of the most severely affected cases do not survive infancy. Individuals who do develop speech often have severe impairments, largely neurologically based. Utterance length is short, dysarthria and dyspraxia are common, and articulation errors caused by hypotonia and compensatory patterns secondary to cleft palate are common.

Feeding Disorders: Early failure-to-thrive is one of the more common manifestations of SLO. Feeding difficulties in infancy are caused by a combination of severe hypotonia, upper airway obstruction, lower airway problems (including pulmonary hypoplasia), congenital heart disease, irritability, and pyloric stenosis. Vomiting is common and has often been mistaken for "reflux."

Hearing Disorders: Specific hearing loss has not typically been associated with SLO, but chronic middle ear disease with resulting transient conductive hearing loss is common.

Voice Disorders: Wet hoarseness secondary to chronic pulmonary disease is common. A "squealing" cry is commonly observed in infancy.

Resonance Disorders: Hypernasality secondary to cleft palate and velopharyngeal insufficiency is to be expected in cases with clefts.

Language Disorders: Language impairment is essentially ubiquitous. In the most severe cases who survive, there may be little or no functional language development. In the mildest cases, language development is usually severely impaired with expressive language usually disproportionately more severely affected than receptive.

Other Clinical Features:

Central nervous system: mental retardation; severe hypotonia; infantile irritability; cortical hypoplasia; cerebellar hypoplasia; absence of the corpus callosum; hydrocephaly;

Growth: small stature;

Craniofacial: cleft palate; micrognathia; microglossia; microcephaly; square, high forehead; short nose with anteverted nostrils; Robin sequence; minor auricular anomalies; thickened alveolar ridges, especially of the maxilla;

Genitourinary: micropenis in males; ambiguous genitalia; cryptorchidism; kidney anomalies; ureter stenosis; hydronephrosis;

Cardiopulmonary: congenital heart anomalies, including tetralogy of Fallot or ventriculoseptal defect; pulmonary hypoplasia; lung malformations;

Gastrointestinal: pyloric stenosis;

Limbs: soft tissue syndactyly of the second and third toes; polydactyly; contractures of the fingers; hip dislocation;

Metabolic: decreased serum cholesterol.

Natural History: Many babies with SLO are born in a breech position. Neonatal death is common in the most severely affected individuals, and death in infancy occurs in an additional 20% of cases. Early demise is most often related to cardiopulmonary disorders. Irritability in infancy is common and may be related to sterol metabolism. Cognitive development is almost always severely impaired, with some patients having moderate impairment.

Treatment Prognosis: Dietary supplementation with increased cholesterol has had some benefit, especially in the neonatal period, by reducing irritability and increasing somatic growth. However, in general, the prognosis for significant improvement in psychomotor development remains poor.

Differential Diagnosis: Polydactyly, irritability, cleft palate, and micrognathia are common in trisomy 13 and trisomy 18, both of which also result in neonatal death. Brain anomalies associated with genital hypoplasia are common in the holoprosencephalic spectrum of disorders.

Sotos Syndrome

Also Known As: Cerebral gigantism

Sotos syndrome is one of the syndromes of accelerated growth and early maturation. The syndrome has an interesting behavioral phenotype with aggressive and maladaptive behaviors common. Some clinicians may be tempted to relate the maladaptive behaviors to the somewhat menacing facial appearance some individuals with Sotos syndrome express.

Major System(s) Affected: Growth; craniofacial; central nervous system; endocrine; cardiac; ocular; musculoskeletal.

Etiology: Autosomal dominant inheritance has been suggested, but a gene has not been mapped or identified.

Speech Disorders: Speech is typically delayed in onset. Mild dysarthria may occur. Articulatory distortions occur secondary to dental spacing anomalies. In adolescence, forced speech may develop in association with aggressive behavior.

Feeding Disorders: Early feeding may be compromised by hypotonia.

Hearing Disorders: Hearing is normal in Sotos syndrome.

Voice Disorders: Voice is low pitched for age, but not for height. Hoarseness is an occasional finding that may be secondary to vocal abuse caused by the aggressive behavior displayed by some patients with Sotos syndrome.

Resonance Disorders: Resonance balance is normal in Sotos syndrome.

Language Disorders: Language development is typically delayed, but not usually to a severe extent.

Other Clinical Features:

> **Growth:** accelerated growth; tall stature; increased span; advanced bone age;

> **Craniofacial:** prognathism, macrocephaly; broad, high forehead; dolicocephaly; al-

veolar ridge prominence; premature dental eruption; vertical maxillary excess; pointed chin;

Central nervous system: hypotonia; delayed psychomotor development; seizures; cognitive impairment;

Endocrine: hypothyroidism or hyperthyroidism;

Cardiac: heart anomalies;

Ocular: strabismus;

Musculoskeletal: kyphoscoliosis;

Other: development of neoplasias.

Natural History: Neonates with Sotos syndrome are large at birth and growth accelerates through infancy and childhood. There may be an early onset of puberty. However, growth slows after the onset of puberty and in many cases, adult height is within normal limits. Early motor development would seem to point toward a more severe developmental delay than the actual final outcome. Most individuals with Sotos syndrome have mild impairment or borderline functioning as adults. The possibility for the development of neoplasias, both malignant and benign, requires careful follow-up as children with Sotos syndrome grow. The onset of maladaptive behaviors coincides with the premature onset of puberty in many cases and becomes progressively worse with the development of impulsive and obsessive behaviors. Obsessive-compulsive disorder has been observed. Aggressiveness can be disturbing in Sotos syndrome because the affected individuals are typically larger than their peers.

Treatment Prognosis: Individuals with Sotos syndrome respond well to speech-language therapy. Overall muscle tone also improves with age.

Differential Diagnosis: Weaver syndrome has very early acceleration of growth, as in Sotos syndrome, but the growth does not abate in **Weaver syndrome.** Like Sotos syndrome, children with **Beckwith-Wiedemann syndrome** have overgrowth, prognathism, propensity toward neoplasias (such as Wilms tumor), and hypotonia. Sotos syndrome does not feature omphalocele or hypoglycemia, as does **Beckwith-Wiedemann syndrome,** and overall facial appearance is different.

Spondyloepiphyseal Dysplasia Congenita

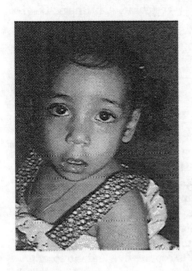

Spondyloepiphyseal dysplasia congenita.

Also Known As: SED; spondyloepiphyseal dysplasia

Spondyloepiphyseal dysplasia congenita is a syndrome of short stature that can lead to Robin sequence because micrognathia and cleft palate are common anomalies associated with the syndrome. The syndrome is caused by a mutation in the COL2A1 gene, the same gene responsible for Stickler syndrome. The Stickler mutation, although in the same gene, is a different mutation in a different exon in the gene.

Major System(s) Affected: Growth; craniofacial; ocular; musculoskeletal; central nervous system.

Etiology: Autosomal dominant inheritance. The gene has been mapped to the long arm of chromosome 12 and has been identified as the COL2A1 gene, a gene responsible for type 2 collagen formation.

Speech Disorders: Articulation is often impaired, in part because of malocclusion, in part because of sensorineural hearing loss, and often related to compensatory substitutions secondary to cleft palate and velopharyngeal insufficiency.

Feeding Disorders: Infant feeding is often impaired by upper airway obstruction and cleft palate leading to failure-to-thrive.

Hearing Disorders: Sensorineural hearing loss is a common finding and is occasionally compounded by a conductive component secondary to chronic middle ear disease.

Voice Disorders: Voice is typically high-pitched.

Resonance Disorders: Hypernasality secondary to cleft palate is common.

Language Disorders: Language development is often normal, but is impaired in the small percentage of cases with cognitive impairment.

Other Clinical Features:

Growth: short stature, short trunk variety;

Craniofacial: micrognathia; cleft palate; flat midface;

Ocular: myopia; retinal detachment;

Musculoskeletal: flattened vertebrae; short neck; cervical spine subluxation; odontoid hypoplasia; kyphoscoliosis; lumbar lordosis; pectus excavatum or carinatum;

Central nervous system: occasional cognitive impairment.

Natural History: Skeletal anomalies are present at birth and growth deficiency becomes obvious early in life. Myopia is often congenital, but may not be detected until later in childhood. The myopia is progressive and vitreoretinal degeneration may result in retinal detachment. Hearing loss may also be progressive, especially in high frequencies.

Treatment Prognosis: The short stature is related to a primary skeletal dysplasia and, because it is of the short trunk variety, treatment is not possible at the present time. There is no contraindication to standard treatment for cleft palate. Feeding disorders can be resolved by treating the respiratory disorder which rarely requires tracheotomy.

Differential Diagnosis: **Diastrophic dysplasia syndrome** is another syndrome of short stature, cleft palate, and Robin sequence. The skeletal abnormalities are different and can be detected by radiographs.

Steinert Syndrome

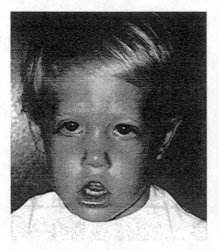 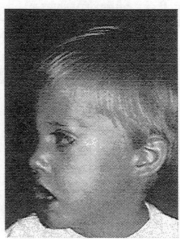

Steinert syndrome: Note myopathic facies, mouth-open posture, and vertical growth pattern.

Also Known As: Myotonic dystrophy

Steinert syndrome is one of the more common forms of muscular dystrophy. The syndrome is interesting in genetic terms because it shows both anticipation and imprinting. Myotonic dystrophy affects all types of muscle (skeletal, smooth, and cardiac) so that speech and swallowing are both potentially impaired. When inherited from the mother, the disorder is expressed at birth and cognitive and language impairment is common.

Major System(s) Affected: Musculoskeletal; central nervous system; craniofacial; integument; ocular, genitourinary; gastrointestinal.

Etiology: Autosomal dominant inheritance. The disorder is one of a number of genetic disorders caused by an expansion of trinucleotide repeats, specifically a series of CTG repeats in a protein kinase gene mapped to 19q13.2-q13.3.

Speech Disorders: In congenital cases (maternally inherited), speech is severely delayed. Oral contacts are extremely weak and oral articulation extremely difficult. Few consonant sounds are recognizable. Lingual movements are severely impaired, and lip incompetence is the rule. In late-onset cases (paternally inherited), early speech development is normal and articulation is normal. Following onset (usually in the second decade of life), articulation may deteriorate, with mild dysarthria and weak oral contacts for pressure consonants.

Feeding Disorders: Feeding impairments with failure-to-thrive occurs only in the congenital form of Steinert syndrome. Swallowing is impaired because of involvement of smooth muscle as well as skeletal muscle. Weak oral movements prevent a lip seal around the nipple with poor or absent suction. Lower intestinal movements are also impaired resulting in constipation and megacolon, thus creating an uncomfortable abdominal feeling and lack of appetite. In addition, muscle tone abnormalities result in upper airway obstruction and there

is reduced pulmonary effort, thus further complicating feeding.

Hearing Disorders: Sensorineural hearing loss is a common clinical manifestation of Steinert syndrome and may be moderate to severe. It is typically progressive.

Voice Disorders: Breathy voice is common in the congenital form. In the late-onset form, voice is initially normal, but may eventually become breathy with progression of the myotonia.

Resonance Disorders: Hypernasality is common in both the congenital and late-onset forms of Steinert syndrome. In the congenital form, hypernasality is often present from the onset of speech. In the late-onset form, the spontaneous development of hypernasality is often the first presenting symptom of myotonic dystrophy. The hypernasality becomes progressively worse with advancement of the disorder.

Language Disorders: In the congenital form, language is delayed and impaired. The degree of impairment is variable, but in the most severe cases, language impairment can be very severe with expressive language more significantly affected than receptive.

Other Clinical Features:

Musculoskeletal: myotonia; progressive muscle wasting; club foot; thin ribs (congenital form);

Central nervous system: polyneuropathy; cognitive impairment (congenital form); personality change (late-onset form);

Craniofacial: vertical facial growth pattern with vertical maxillary excess secondary to lax facial musculature; eyelid ptosis; facial diplegia; Robin sequence (rare, in congenital form only);

Integument: male frontal balding in late onset form;

Ocular: cataracts; lens opacities;

Genitourinary: hypogonadism; urinary tract anomalies;

Gastrointestinal: megacolon; constipation;

Other: malignant hyperthermia in reponse to anesthesia.

Natural History: In the congenital form, the earliest signs of the syndrome are during gestation. Mothers often note reduced fetal movement and may develop polyhydramnios. In the congenital form, muscle weakness is evident immediately and is severe, often with accompanying cognitive impairment and developmental delay. Speech is often the slowest of all developmental milestones. In the late-onset form, the spontaneous development of hypernasality is often one of the earliest findings, usually occurring in early adolescence. The disorder is always progressive.

Treatment Prognosis: All support therapies are indicated in the congenital form, but the more severe the expression, the less positive the response. In the late-onset form, support therapies are also indicated and have a better chance for a positive outcome. Because hypernasality is a common finding, there may be referral for pharyngeal surgery, such as pharyngeal flap. However, many patients with Steinert syndrome respond to general anesthesia with a severe elevation of body temperature (malignant hyperthermia or hyperpyrexia) that can be potentially fatal. However, surgery can be performed successfully if the anesthesiologist is prepared for the complication.

Differential Diagnosis: Muscle weakness and wasting is a common manifestation of many muscular dystrophies. The differential diagnosis is dependent on muscle biopsy to determine the specific enzymatic abnormalities.

S

Stickler Syndrome

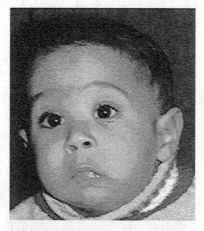
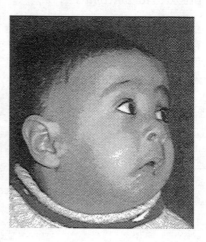
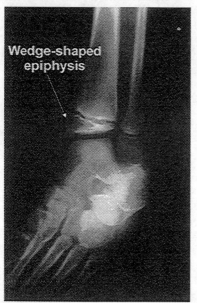

Wedge-shaped
epiphysis

*Stickler syndrome: Note the round
facies, depressed nasal root, and
micrognathia (top row). The
epiphysis at the ankle is wedge-
shaped (bottom).*

Also Known As: Hereditary arthroophthalmopathy

Stickler syndrome is one of the most common connective tissue dysplasias in humans and is the most common syndrome that results in the Robin sequence. At least one-third of all babies initially diagnosed with Robin sequence have Stickler syndrome. The diagnosis can be difficult because most children with Stickler syndrome are normal in appearance, and the minor alterations they express in terms of craniofacial appearance are not particularly stigmatizing. Most children with Stickler syndrome could be called "cute" with round, cherubic faces. However, the syndrome has major impacts on speech, feeding, and hearing. The phenotype of what most clinicians label as Stickler syndrome is probably caused by more than one gene, all involved in the morphogenesis of collagen, a major component of cartilage and connective tissue. Because some skeletal structures are initially cartilaginous, eventual skeletal formation is also affected. The COL2A1, COL11A1, and COL11A2 genes have all been implicated in producing the Stickler phenotype. It is unclear if the phenotypes caused by mutations in these separate genes are exactly the same, or simply close phenocopies.

Major System(s) Affected: Craniofacial; ocular; growth; musculoskeletal.

Etiology: Autosomal dominant inheritance. Several genes have been identified as possibly causing Stickler syndrome, including COL2A1, COL11A1, and COL11A2. COL2A1 has been mapped to 12q13.11-q13.2. The candidate genes for Stickler syndrome are responsible for formation of collagen, a major component of connective tissue and cartilage. Different mutations in this same gene cause spondyloepiphyseal dysplasia congenita and Kniest syndrome.

Speech Disorders: Articulation disorders secondary to malocclusion are common. Micrognathia, with or without anterior skeletal open-bite, is a common finding in Stickler syndrome, resulting in lingual-protrusion distortions. In cases with severe micrognathia, tongue-backing may occur. Compensatory articulation patterns secondary to cleft palate and velopharyngeal insufficiency should be expected in some cases.

S

Feeding Disorders: Early neonatal respiratory distress and upper airway obstruction often lead to feeding disorders. Failure-to-thrive in Stickler syndrome is solely related to upper airway obstruction, often the product of glossoptosis. A short genioglossus muscle and lingual attachment in the mandible restricts anterior tongue movement.

Hearing Disorders: Sensorineural hearing loss, usually in the high frequencies, is found in at least 15% of patients with Stickler syndrome. Conductive loss secondary to chronic middle ear effusion is also seen in cases with cleft palate.

Voice Disorders: Voice production is typically normal in Stickler syndrome.

Resonance Disorders: Hypernasality secondary to cleft palate is an occasional finding. Hyponasality, or cul-de-sac resonance, has also been observed in cases with an extremely small nasal cavity or small nostrils.

Language Disorders: Language development is typically normal in Stickler syndrome, as is cognitive development.

Other Clinical Features:

Craniofacial: micrognathia; cleft palate; Robin sequence; acute angulation of the cranial base; short ramus with normal condyles; antegonial notching of the body of the mandible; maxillary hypoplasia; depressed nasal root; round face; epicanthal folds;

Ocular: myopia, often congenital and severe; vitreoretinal degeneration; retinal detachment resulting in blindness; occasional cataracts;

Growth: occasional short stature; occasional tall stature;

Musculoskeletal: lax joints; epiphyseal dysplasia; osteochondrodysplasia; spondyloepiphyseal dysplasia; joint pains, especially in the knees or lower back.

Natural History: Many babies with Stickler syndrome are born with Robin sequence, constituting approximately one third of all babies with Robin. Micrognathia may be severe at birth resulting in respiratory and feeding disorders with failure-to-thrive. With age, the maxilla and mandible often become proportionate, leading some clinicians to believe that the mandible is exhibiting "catch-up growth." However, the situation is such that the mandible is not really growing so much as the maxilla is hypoplastic. Some children with Stickler syndrome are initially thought to be hypotonic, but in most cases, joint hyperextensibility is related to connective tissue dysplasia rather than true hypotonia.

Treatment Prognosis: Excellent. With proper care, severe eye problems can be avoided. Cleft palate repair is typically successful. Orthognathic surgery is not generally necessary, but is not contraindicated when micrognathia persists.

Differential Diagnosis: Robin sequence and eye problems also occur in **SED congenita** (spondyloepiphyseal dysplasia), but short stature in SED is far more pronounced. **Kniest syndrome,** also caused by a mutation in COL2A1, has a similar facial phenotype, but more severe short stature and marked distortion of the thorax. Isolated (nonsyndromic) Robin sequence has a very similar presentation at birth, but does not have joint or ocular problems as associated findings.

S

Sturge-Weber Syndrome

Also Known As: Sturge-Weber angiomatosis

Sturge-Weber syndrome is an easily recognized, yet still somewhat mysterious, disorder because of the absence of a firm etiologic basis. The syndrome presents with many neurological findings, including seizures, and communicative impairment in the form of speech and language disorders is consistent. The population frequency of the disorder is not known.

Major System(s) Affected: Integument; craniofacial; dental; ocular; central nervous system.

Etiology: Unknown. Autosomal dominant inheritance has been suggested, but all known cases have been spontaneous occurrences.

Speech Disorders: Speech is almost always delayed and always impaired after it develops. Articulation has two major categories of abnormalities: distortions, substitutions, and compensations secondary to oral structural anoma-lies and dysarthria and distortions secondary to central nervous system impairment. Abnormal overgrowth of one side of the face, common in Sturge-Weber syndrome, results in vertical excess of one side of the maxilla, lateral open-bite, and malocclusion. The gingiva may have severe angiomatosis resulting in thickened soft tissue and the underlying overgrowth of the maxillary alveolus may be accompanied by macrodontia. Early dental eruption on the affected side of the face is common. However, dental eruption may also be delayed if the alveolar soft tissues are severely hypertrophic. The common nature of dental eruption abnormalities causes placement errors. The tongue is often thickened on the affected side, also affecting articulation. The neurological abnormalities associated with the syndrome typically result in mild dysarthria and sluggish articulation that may slow the rate of speech.

Feeding Disorders: Feeding disorders have not typically been associated with Sturge-Weber syndrome.

Hearing Disorders: Hearing disorders have not been observed or reported.

Voice Disorders: Hoarseness is an occasional finding in Sturge-Weber syndrome.

Resonance Disorders: Oral resonance is occasionally impaired by the soft tissue overgrowth of the oral cavity.

Language Disorders: Language development is delayed and language is essentially universally impaired secondary to anomalies of the central nervous system.

Other Clinical Features:

Integument: hemangiomas; port wine cutaneous hemangioma of the face;

Craniofacial: unilateral soft tissue and skeletal overgrowth;

Dental: premature dental eruption; occasional delayed dental eruption; macrodontism; malocclusion;

Ocular: choroid hemangiomas; glaucoma;

Central nervous system: arachnoid hemangiomas; leptomeningeal angiomas; vascular anomalies; seizures; cortical calcifications.

Natural History: The angiomas and hemangiomas are present at birth and do not typically progress. The unilateral facial overgrowth is progressive with age, especially in the growth years surrounding eruption of the permanent teeth. Seizures, when present, usually begin in infancy.

Treatment Prognosis: Seizures tend to be difficult to manage and may not respond to normal anticonvulsant medication. Surgery occasionally becomes necessary to remove abnormal vascular regions in the brain.

Differential Diagnosis: Sturge-Weber syndrome is distinctive because of the facial hemangioma. Similar angiomatous lesions may be found in **Klippel-Trénaunay-Weber syndrome.**

S

Treacher Collins Syndrome

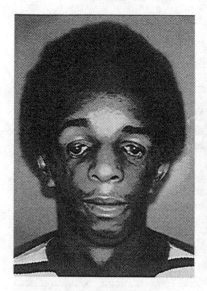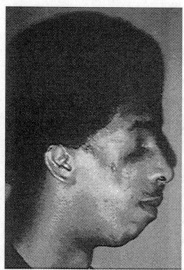

Treacher Collins syndrome: Note the downslanting eyes, malar depressions, micrognathia, and the projection of hair onto the cheek.

Also Known As: mandibulofacial dysostosis; Franceschetti-Klein syndrome, Franceschetti-Zwahlen-Klein syndrome

Treacher Collins syndrome, named for 19th century ophthalmologist Edward Treacher Collins, has been recognized as a distinct multiple anomaly disorder for over 150 years. Although relatively rare, the syndrome has such a distinctive ap-

pearance that it is one of the most easily recognized of craniofacial syndromes. There are no extracranial anomalies associated with Treacher Collins syndrome, although some have been reported. It is likely that some patients have other common anomalies, including congenital heart malformations (such as VSD) in association with the syndrome as a chance and coincidental occurrence. Treacher Collins syndrome is widely regarded as having a population prevalence of 1:10,000. Expression is highly variable, and some affected individuals are quite normal in appearance, while others have severe craniofacial malformations.

Major System(s) Affected: Craniofacial.

Etiology: Autosomal dominant inheritance. The gene has been mapped to 5q32-q33.1 and has been labeled the TREACLE gene.

Speech Disorders: Articulation is commonly impaired in Treacher Collins syndrome in a number of ways. In some cases, the severe micrognathia causes persistent tongue-backing with multiple substitutions for anterior sounds (such as bilabials, lingua-alveolars, and lingua-dentals) with posterior sounds, including compensatory maneuvers such as pharyngeal stops, laryngeal stops, and pharyngeal fricatives. Also common are anterior distortions secondary to anterior skeletal open-bite, a frequent anomaly in the syndrome. Cleft palate, sometimes near absence of the palate, can contribute to additional abnormal compensations, including glottal stops.

Feeding Disorders: Early feeding problems and failure-to-thrive are very common manifestations of Treacher Collins syndrome in the neonatal period and infancy and are related to airway obstruction. Airway obstruction has a number of etiologies, including choanal atresia or stenosis, micrognathia, Robin sequence, and pharyngeal hypoplasia. Babies with Treacher Collins often have severe upper airway obstruction as soon as they close their mouths. Resolution of the airway problems allows normal feeding.

Hearing Disorders: Probably the most common clinical feature of the syndrome is conductive hearing loss. Even patients with very mild facial manifestations of Treacher Collins syndrome have conductive hearing loss. Fixation of the footplate of the stapes is common even when the ossicles and middle ear are intact. Maximal conductive hearing loss is common because Grade II and Grade III microtia are common anomalies. Complete atresia of the middle ear and ossicles is common.

Voice Disorders: Voice is typically normal in Treacher Collins syndrome.

Resonance Disorders: Resonance disorders are very common and unusual in Treacher Collins syndrome. Hypernasality is possible in cases with cleft palate or cleft lip and palate. However, because the entire pharynx is very small in diameter, hypernasality is much less common than hyponasality or mixed resonance. In cases of mixed resonance, it is common to find hyponasality with occasional nasal turbulence and nasal emission. Oral resonance is often severely impaired by retrodisplacement of the tongue and a hypoplastic pharyngeal airway. Oral resonance is muffled with marked damping of sound that would normally resonate in the oropharynx and nasopharynx. Even normal sized tonsils can further impair oral resonance characteristics. Oral resonance and nasal resonance abnormalities are not mutually exclusive and may coexist.

Language Disorders: Language is almost always normal in Treacher Collins syndrome, as is intellect unless there has been severe neonatal hypoxia with subsequent hypoxic brain damage.

Other Clinical Features:

   Craniofacial: downslanting palpebral fissures; clefting or absence of the zygomas; malar bone clefting; bony orbital clefts; micrognathia, often very severe; antegonial notching of the mandible; acute cranial base angle; notch in the lower eyelid; absence of eyelashes on the inner third of the eye; absent puncta; lacrimal duct stenosis or obstruction; microtia; cleft palate; cleft lip and palate (less common than cleft palate alone); projection of hair onto the cheek; absence of angle between the nasal bridge and the forehead; anterior skeletal open-bite.

Natural History: The anomalies associated with Treacher Collins syndrome are all present at birth and there is no progression. Upper airway obstruction may not be obvious initially, but is often present within the first few days of life. In cases with more severe craniofacial manifestations, airway obstruction is immediate after birth.

Treatment Prognosis: All structural anomalies in Treacher Collins syndrome can be treated surgically, and in many cases, outcomes can be very good. Osseous distraction is a new tool being used for severe micrognathia early in life. The palatal clefts can often be difficult to repair because of a severe tissue deficiency, but hypernasality may not be a problem even in cases with severe palatal anomalies. The airway obstruction is so severe in some cases that tracheotomy becomes necessary. Bone conduction hearing aids are indicated in cases with severe microtia, but in less severe microtia, it may be possible to use air conduction aids. Caution needs to be exercised in reconstructive surgery in the middle ear because of an anomalous course of the VIIth cranial nerve, which may course through the footplate of the stapes.

Differential Diagnosis: In the earlier years of the delineation of Treacher Collins syndrome, the disorder was often lumped together with **oculo-auriculo-vertebral dysplasia,** thought to be a unilateral expression of the same disorder. Miller syndrome has similar craniofacial manifestations, but has unusual limb anomalies. Probably most similar to Treacher Collins syndrome is **Nager syndrome. Nager syndrome** has very similar craniofacial anomalies, but also has thumb and radial anomalies not found in Treacher Collins Syndrome.

Turner Syndrome

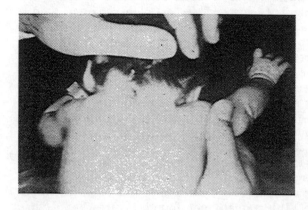

Webbing of the neck in an infant with Turner syndrome.

Also Known As: XO syndrome; 45, X syndrome; monosomy X; Morgagni-Turner-Albright syndrome; Schereshevkii-Turner syndrome; Bonnevie-Ulrich syndrome; Turner-Varny syndrome

Turner syndrome is a relatively common multiple anomaly syndrome, with a population prevalence of approximately 1:2,500. All affected individuals are phenotypically females because the disorder is caused by absence of one of the sex chromosomes leaving a single X chromosome (sex chromosome, or X chromosome monosomy). Many cases are mosaics, meaning that not all of the cells in the body have 45X karytoypes. The larger the percentage of cells that have the missing X

chromosome, the more severe the expression of the disorder. In cases that have 100% of the cells with an X chromosome monosomy, there is absence of secondary sexual characteristics, absence of gonads, and short stature. Webbing of the neck is variable.

Major System(s) Affected: Growth; genitourinary; craniofacial; musculoskeletal; limbs; integument; cardiac; central nervous system; endocrine; ocular.

Etiology: Deletion of one copy of the X chromosome from all or some of the cells in the body.

Speech Disorders: Articulation impairment secondary to malocclusion is common, including lingual protrusion secondary to anterior skeletal open-bite and, in some cases, tongue-backing secondary to micrognathia. Speech onset is often delayed.

Feeding Disorders: Early failure-to-thrive may occur secondary to airway obstruction, micrognathia, and/or Robin sequence.

Hearing Disorders: Sensorineural hearing loss is found in approximately half of individuals with Turner syndrome. In some cases, chronic middle ear disease may result in a mixed loss.

Voice Disorders: Hoarseness is common, as is a high-pitched voice in some cases.

Resonance Disorders: Hypernasality secondary to cleft palate or submucous cleft palate is common.

Language Disorders: Language impairment, especially in terms of expressive language is common, although cognitive impairment is not a common finding in the syndrome. Nearly all patients have normal intellect, but learning disorders are relatively common, usually in the areas of mathematics and spatial relationships. These problems are usually relatively minor.

Other Clinical Features:

Growth: short stature;

Genitourinary: gonadal aplasia (in complete monosomies) or hypoplasia (in mosaicism); kidney anomalies;

Craniofacial: cleft palate (often submucous); micrognathia; malocclusion; epicanthi; low-set posteriorly rotated ears; prominent ears; low posterior hairline;

Musculoskeletal: broad (shield-shaped) chest resulting in wide-spaced nipples; hip dislocation; scoliosis; skeletal dysplaisa;

Limbs: cubitus valgus; spoon-shaped nails; short fourth metatarsal and metacarpal; knee anomalies;

Integument: multiple pigmented nevi; tendency to form keloid scars; webbing of the neck (pterygium coli);

Cardiac: aortic valve anomalies, coarctation of the aorta;

Central nervous system: learning disabilities;

Endocrine: absence or incomplete development of secondary sexual characteristics; diabetes mellitus; thyroid disorders;

Ocular: cataracts; strabismus; ptosis.

Natural History: The major anomalies associated with Turner syndrome are typically evident at birth in cases of complete monosomies. In patients with mosaicisms, anomalies may be minor, almost unnoticeable in many cases. The first indications of the diagnosis in such cases may be primary amenorrhea and delayed or absent development of secondary sexual characteristics. Life expectancy is not known to be impaired.

Treatment Prognosis: Symptomatic treatments are effective, including the use of growth hormone and estrogen replacement. Speech therapy, palatal surgery, and orthognathic surgery are all indicated, as is language therapy in those cases with impairment.

Differential Diagnosis: Noonan syndrome when present in females has many similar features, although the heart anomalies are different. Some patients with velo-cardio-facial syndrome have webbing of the neck together with retrognathia, cleft palate, and mild growth deficiency. Karyotype will differentiate the syndromes.

Van Buchem Syndrome

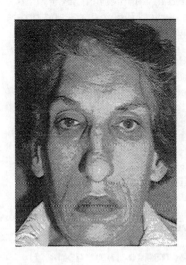

Bony overgrowth of the face in van Buchem syndrome.

Also Known As: van Buchem disease; generalized cortical hyperostosis; hyperphosphatasemia tarda; endosteal hyperostosis; sclerosteosis (thought by some to be the same disorder while other clinicians believe this is a separate, but similar syndrome)

van Buchem syndrome is an autosomal recessive disorder of bony overgrowth that generally shows a late onset of clinical findings, although it is probable that the actual process begins early in life. The disorder has most often been reported in people of Dutch descent, including South Africans of Dutch ancestry. It has been suggested that van Buchem syndrome and a disorder known as sclerosteosis represent the same disorder. Sclerosteosis has also been reported primarily in individuals of Dutch descent, including South Africans (Afrikaners). The skeletal findings in van Buchem syndrome and sclerosteosis are essentially the same, but sclerosteosis has been described as being more severe and involving syndactyly of the second and third fingers. However, these findings may represent variable expression of the same disorder. Therefore, there will not be a separate entry for sclerosteosis.

Major System(s) Affected: Craniofacial; skeletal; central nervous system; ocular.

Etiology: Autosomal recessive inheritance. The gene has been mapped to 17q11.2.

Speech Disorders: Initially, speech is normal. As bony overgrowth becomes more severe, the cranial nerves become compressed. Dysarthria becomes progressive. Prior to the onset of dysarthria, articulation may be impaired by progressive bony overgrowth that results in abnormalities of jaw structure, which may result in malocclusion and obligatory placement errors. Facial parasthesia may exacerbate the problem.

Feeding Disorders: Early feeding is not impaired. Later in life, continuous compression of the cranial nerves, the spinal cord, and brain stem can lead to dysphagia. There is some loss of sensation in the facial musculature.

Hearing Disorders: Progressive hearing loss is a near constant finding. The hearing loss is typically mixed at first, progressing to a pro-found sensorineural hearing loss related to compression of the auditory nerve. Hyperostoses and progressive otosclerosis can also contribute to a moderate to severe conductive component with fixed and fused ossicles common. The onset of hearing loss is typically in the teen years.

Voice Disorders: Voice is initially normal, and then becomes progressively hoarse or breathy with restricted motion of the vocal cords, probably related to progressive sclerosis of the laryngeal cartilages.

Resonance Disorders: Hyponasality secondary to nasal obstruction may develop late in life.

Language Disorders: Language development is normal.

Other Clinical Features:

Craniofacial: progressive enlargement of the mandible with occasional asymmetry, often appearing square at the chin; exorbitism; mild hypertelorism; skeletal overgrowth resulting in closure of the cranial foramina, including the optic foramen and compression of the auditory nerve; thickening of the calvarium; progressive facial paresis;

Skeletal: diaphyseal thickening of the long bones; cortical hyperostosis;

Central nervous system: headaches; progressive increase of intracranial pressure; compression of the cranial nerves; anosmia;

Ocular: progressive optic atrophy; strabismus; occasional blindness.

Natural History: There is significant variability of expression, but in many of the most severe cases, symptoms are evident in infancy, including facial paresis. In milder cases, significant clinical features may not become apparent until the second or third decade of life. The neurological findings and hearing loss are progressive. In the most severe cases, increased intracranial pressure and nerve compression can become life-threatening.

Treatment Prognosis: The progressive nature of the skeletal changes is intractable, but if not severe, the effects on the quality of life may be relatively mild, especially early in the expression of the disorder. Palliative treatment and surgical management are difficult because of the continuous production of new bone. Initial hearing loss will respond well to amplification, but the benefit may eventually be lost.

Differential Diagnosis: Progressive thickening of bone with craniofacial changes is common in the small number of syndromes categorized as osteochondrodysplasias, including craniometaphyseal dysplasia, frontometaphyseal dysplasia, and craniodiaphyseal dysplasia. Each has its own characteristic type of progression and effects on the long bones and cranium so that the diagnosis can be differentiated by radiographic study.

van der Woude Syndrome

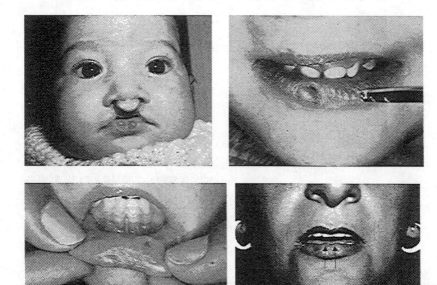

van der Woude syndrome: Infant with bilateral cleft lip and palate with lip pits (upper left). Lip pits on the vermilion surface (upper right) and on the buccal surface of the lower lip (lower left). Lip mounds in an adult (lower right).

Also Known As: Cleft lip and palate with lip pits; cleft lip and palate with mucous cysts of the lower lip; lip pit syndrome

van der Woude syndrome is one of the more common syndromes of clefting. In pedigrees that have mixing of cleft type (some cases with cleft palate only, others with cleft lip or cleft lip and palate), the first suspicion should be van der Woude syndrome unless there are obvious extracranial anomalies consistent with another multiple anomaly disorder. van der Woude syndrome has been estimated to have a population prevalence of 1:35,000 people, constituting approximately 2% of all people with clefts. This estimate is probably low because the syndrome has very few associated anomalies and may be expressed without the presence of lip pits. Thus, it is possible for someone to express the autosomal dominant gene for van der Woude syndrome and have a cleft lip and palate, but no anomalies of the lower lip. Conversely, some individuals have lip pits or mounds without clefting. It is more likely that 4–5% of patients at cleft palate centers have van der Woude syndrome so that the population prevalence may be closer to 1:15,000.

Major System(s) Affected:
Craniofacial/oral.

Etiology:
Autosomal dominant inheritance. The gene has been mapped to 1q32.

Speech Disorders:
Speech onset is normal. Articulation may be impaired by compensatory articulation patterns secondary to cleft palate and velopharyngeal insufficiency. In cases with cleft lip and alveolus, obligatory anterior distortions are likely.

Feeding Disorders:
Feeding disorders are not typically encountered, but cleft palate may complicate early efforts to feed in the neonatal period.

Hearing Disorders:
Conductive hearing loss secondary to chronic serous otitis is found in 70–75% of patients with van der Woude syndrome.

Voice Disorders:
Voice is typically normal.

Resonance Disorders:
Hypernasality is possible secondary to cleft palate. A slightly flat cranial base (platybasia) may be a factor in causing a slightly higher frequency of velopharyngeal insufficiency in van der Woude syndrome than in individuals with isolated clefts.

Language Disorders:
Language is normal in van der Woude syndrome.

Other Clinical Features:

Craniofacial/oral: cleft lip; cleft palate; pits or mounds (cysts) of the lower lip or on the buccal surface of the lower lip; ankyloglossia; mild platybasia; higher than normal frequency of congenitally missing permanent premolars in both the maxillary and mandibular arches.

Natural History: All of the anomalies are present at birth. The lip pits may occasionally secrete saliva because they are connected to small salivary glands. When large, the pits may occasionally trap small food particles resulting in infection.

Most often, the pits are too small for this to occur.

Treatment Prognosis: All of the anomalies in van der Woude syndrome may be treated effectively with reconstructive surgery.

Differential Diagnosis: Popliteal pterygium syndrome also has clefting and lower lip pits as common features, but also has other limb anomalies and a tendency toward significant midfacial hypoplasia.

Velo-Cardio-Facial Syndrome (VCFS)

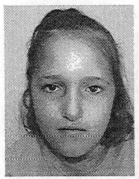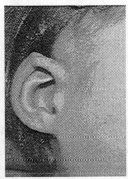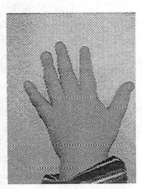

Velo-cardio-facial syndrome: Characteristic appearance of the face, showing a vertically long face, pear-shaped nose, overfolded helices on the ears with attached lobules (center), and small hands with tapered digits (right).

Also Known As: DiGeorge sequence (DGS); Cayler syndrome; conotruncal anomalies face syndrome; Sedlačková syndrome; 22q11 deletion syndrome; CATCH 22 (*Note:* Although this term has been applied by some clinicians, it has a pejorative connotation in its attempt at humor and should be avoided as a diagnostic label.)

Velo-cardio-facial syndrome (VCFS) is probably the second most com-mon multiple anomaly syndrome in humans with an estimated pop-ulation prevalence of 1:2,000 peo-ple and a birth incidence that is undoubtedly higher because some babies do not survive the neonatal period. VCFS has perhaps the most expansive phenotype of any multi-ple anomaly syndrome with over 180 clinical features already de-scribed. The syndrome was initially delineated because of the associa-tion of congenital heart disease, severe hypernasality, and learning disabilities. A small interstitial chromosomal deletion from the long arm of chromosome 22 at the q11.2 band was identified in 1992 at the same time psychiatric disorders became delineated as a common feature of the syndrome. Some type of communicative disorder is present in nearly all cases, including hypernasality, articulation impairment, language disorders, voice disorders, and conductive, sensorineural, or mixed hearing loss. It has been estimated that at least 5% of all patients in cleft palate clinics have this syndrome.

Major System(s) Affected:
Heart, vascular, craniofacial, central nervous system, skeletal, renal, immune, metabolic, limb, mental, cognitive, digestive, respiratory, genitourinary.

Etiology: A deletion of a small segment of the long arm of chromosome 22 at the 22q11.2 band occurs in the large majority of cases. The deletion is typically nearly 3 million base pairs in length, which encompasses many genes, but it is still not known if the syndrome is a contiguous gene or single gene deletion syndrome. The expression of the syndrome is inherited in an autosomal dominant manner with essentially 100% penetrance. No imprinting or anticipation has been noted. The syndrome is inherited in an autosomal dominant manner.

Speech Disorders: Severe articulation impairment, usually characterized by gross glottal stop substitutions when velopharyngeal insufficiency is present; velopharyngeal insufficiency (usually severe).

Feeding Disorders: There is often copious nasal regurgitation during feeding in the neonatal period which may persist into early childhood. Although pH probes will register strongly positive, this finding should not be confused with "reflux." Classic gastroesophageal reflux does occur in some older children with VCFS, but the problem in infancy is significant emesis. Because of the combined effects of hypotonia and retrognathia, airway obstruction may also occur during feeding which will compromise efforts to nurse efficiently.

Hearing Disorders: Conductive hearing loss secondary to middle ear effusion; occasional sensorineural hearing loss, most often unilateral and mild to moderate, but occasionally severe or profound and occasionally bilateral;

exaggerated startle response and phobic reaction to loud noises, but probably not hyperacusis.

Voice Disorders: High-pitched voice; hoarseness; breathiness.

Resonance Disorders: Hypernasality (usually severe).

Language Disorders: Language impairment (usually mild delay) with marked catch-up in language development between 3 and 4 years of age.

Other Clinical Features:

Craniofacial: platybasia (flat skull base); asymmetric crying facies in infancy; structurally asymmetric face; functionally asymmetric face; vertical maxillary excess (long face); straight facial profile; congenitally missing teeth; small teeth; enamel hypoplasia (primary dentition); hypotonic flaccid facies; downturned oral commissures; cleft lip (uncommon); microcephaly; small posterior cranial fossa;

Optic: tortuous retinal vessels; suborbital congestion ("allergic shiners"); strabismus; narrow palpebral fissures; posterior embryotoxin; small optic disk; prominent corneal nerves; cataract; iris nodules; iris coloboma (uncommon); retinal coloboma (uncommon); small eyes; mild orbital hypertelorism; mild orbital dystopia; puffy eyelids;

Hearing: overfolded helix; attached auricular lobules; protuberant cup-shaped ears; small ears; mildly asymmetric ears; ear tags or pits (uncommon); narrow external ear canals;

Nasal: prominent nasal bridge; bulbous nasal tip; mildly separated nasal domes (appearing bifid); pinched alar base; narrow nostrils;

Cardiovascular: VSD (ventricular septal defect); ASD (atrial septal defect); pulmonic atresia or stenosis; tetralogy of Fallot; right-sided aorta; truncus arteriosus; PDA (patent ductus arteriosus); interrupted aorta; coarctation of the aorta; aortic valve anomalies; aberrant subclavian arteries; vascular ring; anomalous origin of carotid artery; transposition of the great vessels; tricuspid atresia; medially displaced internal carotid arteries; tortuous, kinked, absent, or accessory internal carotids; jugular vein anomalies; absence of vertebral artery (unilateral); low bifurcation of common carotid; tortuous or kinked vertebral arteries; Reynaud's phenomenon; small veins;

Central nervous system: circle of Willis anomalies; periventricular cysts (mostly at anterior horns); small cerebellar vermis; cerebellar hypoplasia/dysgenesis; white matter hyperintensities on MR examination; generalized hypotonia; seizures; strokes; spina bifida/meningomyelocele; mild developmental delay; enlarged Sylvian fissure;

Craniofacial-oral: upper airway obstruction in infancy; absent or small adenoids; laryngeal web (anterior); large pharyngeal airway; laryngomalacia; arytenoid hyperplasia; pharyngeal hypotonia; asymmetric pharyngeal movement; thin pharyngeal muscle; unilateral vocal cord paresis;

Renal: hypoplastic, aplastic, or cystic kidneys;

Digestive: Hirschsprung aganglionic megacolon has been reported in several cases; inguinal hernias; umbilical hernias; malrotation of the bowel; diaphragmatic hernia has been found in several cases; anal anomalies (displaced, imperforate);

Skeletal: small hands and feet; tapered digits; short fingernails and toenails; rough, red, scaly skin on hands and feet; morphea; finger contractures; triphalangeal thumbs; polydactyly (both preaxial and postaxial); soft tissue syndactyly, especially of toes 2 and 3;

Feeding: feeding difficulty; failure-to-thrive; nasal vomiting; gastroesophageal reflux; nasal regurgitation; irritability; chronic constipation;

Cognitive: learning disabilities (math concept, reading comprehension, problem-solving) with concrete thinking and difficulty with abstraction; occasional mild mental retardation; ADD or ADHD; thrombocytopenia; Bernard-Soulier disease; juvenile rheumatoid arthritis;

Mental: mental illness, usually bipolar affective disorder, with rapid or ultrarapid cycling of mood disorder; schizoaffective disorder; impulsiveness; flat affect; dysthymia, cyclothymia; social immaturity; obsessive compulsive disorder; generalized anxiety disorder; phobias;

Respiratory: frequent upper respiratory infections; frequent lower airway disease (pneumonia, bronchitis); reduced T cell populations; reduced thymic hormone; reactive airway disease or asthma;

Genitourinary: hypospadias; cryptorchidism; urethral reflux; hypocalcemia;

Immune: hypoparathyroidism; pseudohypoparathyroidism; hypothyroidism; mild growth deficiency, relative small stature; absent or hypoplastic thymus; hypoplastic pituitary gland;

Skeletal: scoliosis; hemivertebrae; spina bifida occulta; butterfly vertebrae; fused vertebrae (mostly cervical); tethered spinal cord; syrinx; osteopenia; Sprengel anom-

aly; talipes equinovarus (club foot); small skeletal muscles; joint dislocations; chronic leg pains; flat foot arches; hyperextensible and lax joints; extra ribs; rib fusion;

Other: abundant scalp hair; thin appearing skin (venous patterns easily visible); Robin sequence; DiGeorge sequence; Potter sequence; occasional CHARGE association.

Natural History: Early development of children with VCFS is marked by mild delay, with expressive language often showing a slightly larger lag than other milestones. Velopharyngeal insufficiency is common and usually leads to gross glottal stop subsitutions which makes speech largely unintelligible. However, children with VCFS often show a dramatic spurt in development between 3 and 4 years of age. Early cognition is usually within normal limits, but learning disabilities involving abstraction and problem solving become evident in primary school and may be accompanied by a drop in IQ score, especially on performance scales. School performance may be normal in early grades and deteriorate as the learning disorders become more obvious and subject matter becomes more difficult. Attention disorders may become evident in childhood, but often do not respond well to stimulants such as methylphenidate or dexedrine. Onset of psychiatric disorders often occurs in adolescence or young adult life, although childhood psychiatric illness has been reported in some cases. Chronic respiratory and middle ear infections are most severe in early childhood (2 to 5 years of age) and gradually diminish in later childhood years.

Treatment Prognosis: A combination of speech therapy and surgical reconstruction of the velopharyngeal valve can result in normal speech in most cases. Learning problems respond best to repeated drill which is also most effective during speech therapy. Psychiatric problems may progress in adult years to the point of psychosis.

Differential Diagnosis: There are many multiple syndromes with the combination of heart anomalies and cleft palate, including **Niikawa-Kuroki syndrome** (Kabuki makeup syndrome), **fetal alcohol syndrome,** and **CHARGE association.** There are also facial similarities between VCFS and **Langer-Giedion syndrome.** Mild orbital hypertelorism may occur in VCFS which, when in association with hypospadias and feeding difficulties, may lead clinicians to suspect **Opitz syndrome** (the G/BBB syndrome) which is an X-linked disorder. However, the large number of potential anomalies in VCFS can lead clinicians to search for additional phenotypic features prior to requesting FISH studies.

Weaver Syndrome

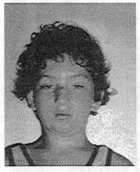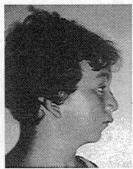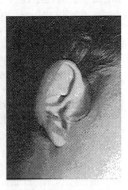

Micrognathia and protuberant ears in Weaver syndrome.

Also Known As: Weaver-Smith Syndrome

Weaver syndrome is one of a small number of overgrowth syndromes that include disorders such as **Sotos syndrome** and **Beckwith-Wiedemann syndrome.** Syndromes of overgrowth are far fewer in number than syndromes of short stature. Therefore, the identification of overgrowth syndromes is somewhat easier with fewer alternative diagnoses.

Major System(s) Affected: Growth; musculoskeletal; central nervous system; craniofacial; limbs; integument; genital.

Etiology: The etiology of Weaver syndrome is still uncertain, but autosomal dominant inheritance is possible, if not likely. No gene has been mapped or identified.

Speech Disorders: Delayed onset of speech is a near constant. Articulation impairment is common, primarily related to hypotonia with sluggish movements of the articulators. Micrognathia also adds a Class II malocclusion to further complicate articulatory placment. A chronic mouth open posture can predispose individuals with Weaver syndrome to lingual protrusion.

Feeding Disorders: Early feeding problems are very common and are typically related to low muscle tone. Mild upper airway obstruction may also occur caused by the combined effects of hypotonia and micrognathia. However, the majority of early feeding problems are related to the central nervous system rather than structural craniofacial anomalies.

Hearing Disorders: Hearing is typically normal in Weaver syndrome.

Voice Disorders: In infancy, the cry of babies with Weaver syndrome is typically low-pitched and hoarse. Voice remains low-pitched, although not necessarily inappropriate for body size.

Resonance Disorders: Hypernasality secondary to velopharyngeal insufficiency caused by hypotonia has been observed.

Language Disorders: Language is always delayed and impaired. Expressive and receptive language are both affected equally.

Other Clinical Features:

   Growth: tall stature;

   Musculoskeletal: early skeletal maturation; lax joints; scoliosis; inguinal and umbilical hernias;

   Central nervous system: developmental delay; hypotonia; spasticity; seizures; cognitive impairment; dilated ventricles;

   Craniofacial: micrognathia; macrocephaly; broad forehead; mild hypertelorism; large ears; prominent chin, often with a midline crease; long, prominent philtrum;

   Limbs: camptodactyly; short small fingers with clinodactyly; thick finger pads; broad thumbs; deep-set fingernails;

   Integument: loose skin; sparse hair;

   Genital: cryptorchidism.

Natural History: Size at birth is usually large. Growth then accelerates and continues unabated even after puberty. Adult height is exceptionally large. Muscle tone is typically low throughout life. The appetite is usually very vigorous, but it would seem that the increase in eating capacity is related to the need for calories to support excessive growth.

Treatment Prognosis: Patients with Weaver syndrome make good progress with symptomatic treatment, including speech, physical, and occupational therapy. The total degree of achievement is predicted most by the degree of cognitive deficiency.

Differential Diagnosis: Sotos syndrome is similar to Weaver syndrome in early life with regard to growth acceleration and bone maturation. However, the craniofacial appearance and behavioral phenotypes vary considerably.

Wildervanck Syndrome

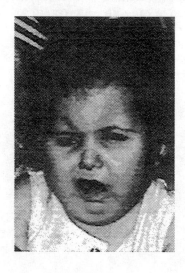

Wildervanck syndrome: Note facial asymmetry.

Also Known As: Cervicooculo-acoustic syndrome

Wildervanck syndrome is an underrecognized disorder that has facial asymmetry, spinal anomalies, hearing loss, and respiratory compromise as consistent clinical features. The disorder could be confused for **oculo-auriculo-vertebral dysplasia** because of the phenotypic overlap.

Major System(s) Affected: Craniofacial; ocular; musculoskeletal; neurologic; growth.

Etiology: Autosomal dominant inheritance. The gene has not been mapped or identified.

Speech Disorders: Speech disorders are highly variable, ranging from severe delay and impairment to essentially normal speech. Speech is affected by sensorineural hearing loss, malocclusion, airway compromise, and cognitive impairment, none of which are constant findings in the syndrome, nor are they mutually exclusive. Normal intellect is the norm in the syndrome, but cognitive impairment has been observed. Posterior airway obstruction can cause fronting and tongue protrusion during speech. Malocclusion secondary to facial asymmetry and occasional anterior skeletal open-bite (growth changes caused by airway obstruction) result in obligatory placement errors and distortions.

Feeding Disorders: Infant and early childhood feeding can be severely compromised by airway obstruction caused by a small pharyngeal airway and retrognathia with a short neck that reduces the vertical dimensions of the airway. Failure-to-thrive may result from airway obstruction, but will resolve with management of the airway disorder. Limited oral opening in some cases may further exacerbate the problem.

Hearing Disorders: Sensorineural and mixed hearing loss are common findings.

Voice Disorders: Voice may be hoarse secondary to chronic airway obstruction causing the lymphoid tissue, even when normal in size, to crowd the pharynx and increase the amount of congestion.

Resonance Disorders: Both hyponasality and hypernasality

have been observed. Hyponasality is secondary to obstruction of an already small airway by the adenoids and/or tonsils. Hypernasality has been observed by the author in a single case that had a submucous cleft palate. Oral resonance is also severely impaired by the combination of a small pharyngeal airway and a vertically short airway. Oral resonance is often muffled.

Language Disorders: Language development is usually normal, but in cases with cognitive impairment, language will be delayed.

Other Clinical Features:

Craniofacial: craniofacial asymmetry; variable external ear anomalies; maxillary and mandibular hypoplasia; acute angulation of the cranial base; low-set, posteriorly rotated ears; low posterior hairline; cleft palate or submucous cleft palate;

Ocular: unilateral or bilateral Duane syndrome (abducens palsy);

Musculoskeletal: cervical spine malformations, including Klippel-Feil anomaly, vertebral fusions, and spina bifida occulta; Sprengel shoulder; torticollis;

Neurologic: occasional cognitive impairment;

Growth: occasional short stature.

Natural History: All anomalies are present at birth, including the hearing loss, and are nonprogressive.

Treatment Prognosis: With proper management of the hearing loss and airway obstruction, the prognosis is generally good. Eventual craniofacial reconstruction can eliminate the malocclusion, but must be deferred until teen years. However, mandibular distraction is probably applicable to the disorder and may also have a positive effect on airway obstruction.

Differential Diagnosis: Oculo-auriculo-vertebral dysplasia has many of the same phenotypic features as Wildervanck syndrome, including spinal anomalies, external ear anomalies, hearing loss (usually conductive), and facial asymmetry. Sensorineural hearing loss with external ear anomalies is found in **BOR syndrome.** However, the Klippel-Feil anomaly and Duane palsy will differentiate Wildervanck syndrome.

Williams Syndrome

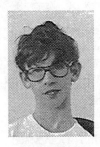

Also Known As: Williams-Beuren syndrome, elfin facies with hypercalcemia

Williams syndrome is one of the more easily recognizable syndromes with a birth frequency of approximately 1:10,000 to 1:15,000. Williams syndrome has particular interest for speech-language pathologists because of its unique language phenotype. Children with Williams syndrome, essentially all of whom are mentally retarded, have very sophisticated language structure.

Major system(s) affected: Central nervous system; craniofacial; dental; cardiac; growth; musculoskeletal; genitourinary; gastrointestinal; endocrine.

Etiology: Interstitial deletion from the long arm of chromosome 7 at 7q11.2 encompassing the elastin gene, labeled as ELN.

Speech Disorders: Articulation may be slightly slurred, and speech rate is often rapid, sometimes causing mild unintelligibility. However, in many cases, articulation skills are quite good with normal intelligibility.

Feeding Disorders: Early failure-to-thrive is common in Williams syndrome and is often attributed to hypotonia and heart anomalies.

Hearing Disorders: Hearing loss is not a primary feature of Williams syndrome, although chronic middle ear effusion has been reported with associated temporary conductive hearing loss. Hyperacusis has been reported as a common finding in Williams syndrome.

Voice Disorders: Voice is often harsh and hoarse.

Resonance Disorders: Resonance is normal.

Language Disorders: Developmental delay is nearly always present with many affected individuals being mildly or moderately retarded, others having borderline normal intellect. When language develops, there is an abundant use of echolalia and clichés. The structure of language use is sophisticated, but the content of the message is often difficult to extract and sometimes makes little sense. Syntax is often impaired. Manner and affect are best described as affable and very interactive, but is accompanied by hyperactivity and impulsivity with poor behavioral control.

Other Clinical Features

Central nervous system: hypotonia, cognitive impairment, strokes, seizures, ADD and ADHD;

Craniofacial: thick lips; long philtrum; anteverted nostrils; epicanthal folds; puffy periorbital area; flaring of the eyebrows; wide mouth;

Dental: hypodontia; microdontia;

Cardiac: supravalvular aortic stenosis; mitral valve prolapse; atrial septal defect; ventriculoseptal defect; pulmonary stenosis;

Growth: short stature;

Musculoskeletal: rib anomalies; limitation of joints; scoliosis; inguinal hernia;

Genitourinary: urinary tract infections; kidney anomalies; urethral stenosis;

Gastrointestinal: chronic constipation; diverticulosis;

Endocrine: hypercalcemia.

Natural History: Developmental milestones are universally delayed, and many infants with Williams syndrome are irritable. In childhood, they become overly friendly and often crave the attention of adults and other children. Although the large majority are cognitively impaired, their sophisticated language structure often makes their performance seem better than it truly is. Many children and adults with Williams syndrome have a strong affinity for music and some have been labeled as "savants" because they often have strong memories for music, names, and facts. Life expectancy is not impaired unless heart anomalies or other vascular structural defects are severe.

Treatment Prognosis: Children with Williams syndrome can learn and they do not have the same "plateau" effect as is seen in Down syndrome. Many of the more severely retarded individuals may require a sheltered or semi-sheltered environment, but others with higher cognitive function can be relatively independent.

Differential Diagnosis: The phenotype of Williams syndrome is distinctive and is not easily confused with other disorders.

Wolf-Hirschhorn Syndrome

Also Known As: del(4p) syndrome; Wolf syndrome

Wolf-Hirschhorn syndrome was initially delineated as a chromosomal deletion syndrome because the first detected cases had large chromosome rearrangements, specifically the deletion of a large segment of the short arm of chromosome 4. More recently, it has been found that the syndrome can be expressed with much smaller rearrangments of chromosome 4, including submicroscopic deletions.

Major System(s) Affected: Central nervous system; growth; craniofacial; ocular; cardiac; genitourinary; gastrointestinal.

Etiology: Deletion of a portion of the short arm of chromosome 4. A large number of cases, well over 10%, are related to translocations in the paternal chromosome 4.

Speech Disorders: There is variability of speech production abnormalities, depending in part on the size of the deletion. In more severe cases, speech does not develop at all. In milder cases, speech onset is delayed and articulation errors are common, related to malocclusion (including disorders related to micrognathia) and cleft anomalies. Compensatory and obligatory errors secondary to clefting may occur.

Feeding Disorders: Early feeding disorder and failure-to-thrive are common in the more severely affected cases related to severe neurological dysfunction and seizures.

Hearing Disorders: Conductive hearing impairment secondary to chronic otitis media in cases with cleft is probable, but other types of hearing loss have not been documented.

Voice Disorders: Early cry is weak.

Resonance Disorders: Hypernasal resonance is common in cases with cleft palate or cleft lip and palate.

Language Disorders: Language disorders vary from complete absence of language development to mild to moderate language impairment.

Other Clinical Features:

Central nervous system: cognitive impairment; seizures; agenesis of the corpus callosum;

Growth: short stature;

Craniofacial: "Greek helmet" facies; prominent nasal root; micrognathia; downturned oral commissures; cleft palate plus/minus cleft lip; low set, featureless ears; microcephaly; hypertelorism; hemangioma; downslanting eyes; scalp defect;

Ocular: iris coloboma; strabismus;

Cardiac: ventriculoseptal defect;

Genitourinary: renal anomalies; hypospadias;

Gastrointestinal: diaphragmatic hernia.

Natural History: All anomalies are present at birth. The developmental and cognitive impairments are global and are accompanied by a generally affectionate and happy temperament.

Treatment Prognosis: The prognosis is dependent on the severity of the cognitive impairment. For example, repairing a palatal cleft makes little sense if the cognitive impairment is so severe as to prevent the development of speech.

Differential Diagnosis: The early presentation, including the weak cry, is similar to **cri-du-chat syndrome.** Karyotype easily differentiates the disorders. Iris coloboma may be associated with **cat eye syndrome, CHARGE association,** and **holoprosencephaly,** all of which may have developmental delay as an associated finding.

X-Linked Mental Retardation

Also Known As: Fragile X syndrome; fragile site mental retardation; Martin-Bell syndrome; marker X syndrome

Probably best known as fragile X syndrome, the label "fragile" refers to early findings from karyotypes that showed a tendency for the X chromosomes of affected individuals to break at a specific site on the long arm when the cell cultures were grown in a folate deficient medium. However, not all individuals with X-linked mental retardation had karyotypes that showed this type of chromosome breakage. In addition, the name "fragile X" implies that the chromosome fragility is in some way responsible for the expression of the disorder, which is not true. The syndrome is one of the most common malformation syndromes in humans with a frequency of 1:2,000 males and a smaller number of affected females so that the total population prevalence is probably between 1:3,000 and 1:4,000.

Major System(s) Affected: Central nervous system; genitals; craniofacial; musculoskeletal; growth; integument.

Etiology: X-linked inheritance. The gene has been mapped to Xq27.3 and has been labeled as FMR1. The mutation is known to be an expansion of a series of trinucleotide repeat sequences (specifically CGG repeats). Normal individuals typically have 6 to 50 of these CGG repeats, but individuals affected with X-linked mental retardation have more than 200 CGG repeats. Some individuals have a "premutation" number of repeats (50 to 200) that predispose the next generation to full manifestation of the syndrome, a process known as *anticipation.* Of females who have the full mutation (over 200 repeats) on one X chromosome, approximately two thirds exhibit some cognitive impairment, with 50% expressing the disorder showing mental retardation and 50% showing borderline intellect but significant learning problems and language impairment. The remaining third have normal intellect.

Speech Disorders: Speech is always impaired in affected males. The onset of speech is delayed, and in many cases, is characterized by persistent echolalia, jargon, dyspraxia, and dysarthria. Some have

428

described the pattern as "cluttering." Anterior articulatory distortions are common and are caused by malocclusion (mandibular prognathism) and dental anomalies. In a small percentage of cases, cleft palate or submucous cleft palate may lead to compensatory articulation substitutions.

Feeding Disorders: In some cases, early hypotonia may complicate feeding, but failure-to-thrive is not one of the hallmarks of the syndrome.

Hearing Disorders: Hearing is typically normal.

Voice Disorders: Hoarseness has been observed in some cases, but this has not been linked to any specific laryngeal anomalies. Some young children have a high-pitched voice.

Resonance Disorders: Hypernasality may occur in cases with cleft palate.

Language Disorders: Language impairment is more severe than the degree of cognitive impairment might predict in many cases. Echolalia and jargon are commonly used, and utterances are often off the subject and nonsensical. Affected individuals often talk to themselves, frequently muttering in a low volume monotonous voice without significant inflection. Utterances are often telegraphic. The number and frequency of gestures are also reduced. Language usage is similar to that seen in many individuals with autism. In the most severe cases, there is limited or absent language usage.

Other Clinical Features:

> **Central nervous system:** mental retardation;
>
> **Genitals:** macroorchidism;
>
> **Craniofacial:** mandibular prognathism; large auricles; broad forehead; thick lips; craniofacial asymmetry; macrocephaly; dental anomalies; occasional cleft palate, often submucous;
>
> **Musculoskeletal:** joint hyperextensibility; scoliosis;
>
> **Growth:** occasional early overgrowth;
>
> **Integument:** hyperpigmentation of the scrotum; periorbital hyperpigmentation.

Natural History: Developmental delay is evident early in infancy. Later, speech and language milestones are severely impaired and many patients develop autisticlike behaviors. A substantial percentage of children given the diagnosis of autism have X-linked mental retardation. An increase in testicular size is observed in childhood, prior to the normal increase at puberty. In childhood, behavior is often difficult to control, including hyperactivity, self-injurious behaviors, and repetitive behaviors such as hand-flapping. Such behaviors often improve after puberty.

Treatment Prognosis: The prognosis is dependent on the degree of cognitive impairment. Intellectual impairment is variable, usually moderate to severe, although often milder in affected females. In the more mildly affected cases, individuals are responsive to speech and language therapy. In the most severe cases, the prognosis for speech and language improvement is poor.

Differential Diagnosis: The facial appearance is sometimes similar to that seen in **Coffin-Lowry syndrome** (coarse facies with prominent lips), **FG syndrome** (prominent lips, prominent forehead), **Beckwith-Wiedemann syndrome** (mandibular prognathism), and **Niikawa-Kuroki syndrome** (large ears).

Index

H